THE POWER OF THE GUT-BRAIN CONNECTION

THE POWER OF THE GUT-BRAIN CONNECTION

HOW TO LEVERAGE THE GUT-BRAIN AXIS TO IMPROVE YOUR PHYSICAL, MENTAL AND EMOTIONAL WELL-BEING

NATASHA HARLOW

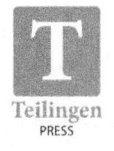

Teilingen
PRESS

Copyright © 2024 by Natasha Harlow

All rights reserved. No part of this book may be reproduced, stored in a retrieval system, or transmitted in any form or by any means, electronic, mechanical, photocopying, recording, or otherwise, without the prior written permission of the publisher, Teilingen Press.

The information contained in this book is based on the author's personal experiences and research. While every effort has been made to ensure the accuracy of the information presented, the author and publisher cannot be held responsible for any errors or omissions.

This book is intended for general informational purposes only and is not a substitute for professional medical, legal, or financial advice. If you have specific questions about any medical, legal, or financial matters matters, you should consult with a qualified healthcare professional, attorney, or financial advisor.

Teilingen Press is not affiliated with any product or vendor mentioned in this book. The views expressed in this book are those of the author and do not necessarily reflect the views of Teilingen Press.

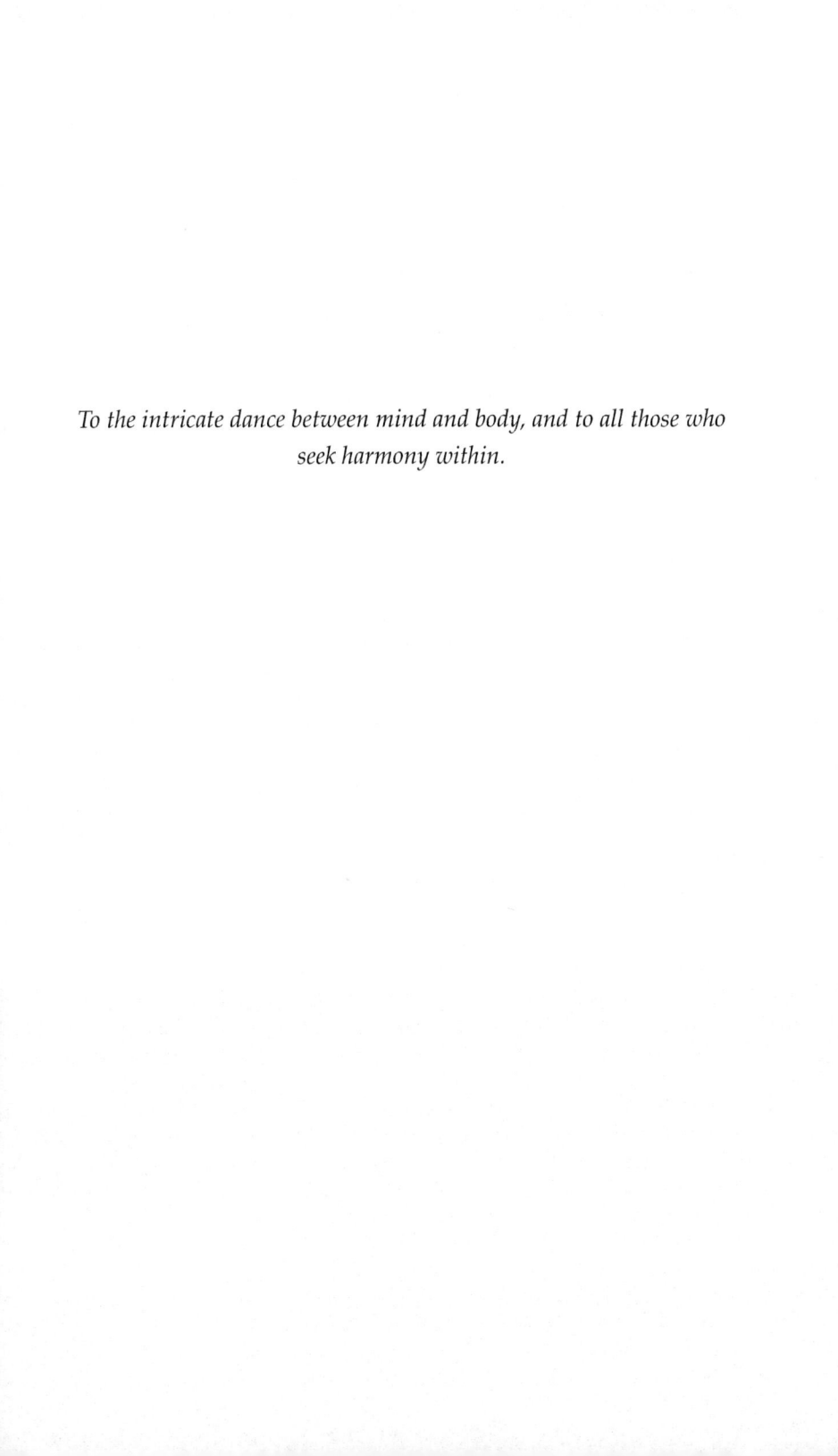

To the intricate dance between mind and body, and to all those who seek harmony within.

Trust your gut. Your gut feelings are usually accurate and correct. If you truly listen to your gut, it can lead you to the life you're meant to live.

OPRAH WINFREY

CONTENTS

Understanding the Gut-Brain Connection   xiii

1. THE SCIENCE OF THE GUT-BRAIN CONNECTION   1
   Neurotransmitters and Hormones   2
   The Role of the Microbiome   3
   Research and Evidence   5
   Challenges and Limitations   6
   Chapter Summary   8

2. DIET AND THE GUT-BRAIN CONNECTION   9
   Foods to Favor   10
   Foods to Avoid   13
   Probiotics and Prebiotics   15
   Dietary Plans and Recommendations   16
   Case Studies   18
   Chapter Summary   19

3. STRESS, EMOTIONS, AND THE GUT   21
   Managing Stress for Gut Health   23
   Mindfulness and Meditation   25
   Therapeutic Approaches   26
   Chapter Summary   27

4. EXERCISE AND THE GUT-BRAIN AXIS   29
   Types of Exercise for Gut Health   30
   Exercise and Gut Flora   32
   Challenges in Starting an Exercise Routine   33
   Maintaining Motivation   35
   Case Studies   36
   Chapter Summary   37

5. SLEEP AND THE GUT-BRAIN CONNECTION   39
   Sleep Disorders and Gut Health   40
   The Role of Circadian Rhythms   41

Practical Tips for Better Sleep and Gut Health	42
Case Studies	45
Chapter Summary	46
6. HOLISTIC APPROACHES TO GUT HEALTH	47
Herbal Remedies and Supplements	48
Acupuncture	50
Massage Therapy	51
Yoga	52
Chapter Summary	53
7. MENTAL HEALTH AND THE GUT	55
The Role of Inflammation	56
Preventative Measures	57
Case Studies	59
Chapter Summary	61
8. CHILDREN AND THE GUT-BRAIN CONNECTION	63
Dietary Impacts on Children	65
Behavioral Issues and the Gut	66
Parental Guidance and Support	67
Case Studies	69
Chapter Summary	70
9. AGING AND THE GUT-BRAIN AXIS	73
Cognitive Decline and the Microbiome	74
Nutritional Needs as We Age	75
Lifestyle Adjustments	77
Case Studies	78
Chapter Summary	79
10. CHRONIC CONDITIONS AND THE GUT-BRAIN CONNECTION	81
Autoimmune Diseases	82
Gastrointestinal Disorders	83
Holistic Management Approaches	84
Case Studies	85
Chapter Summary	86

11. THE FUTURE OF GUT-BRAIN RESEARCH	89
Innovative Research Methods	90
Potential Breakthroughs	92
The Role of Technology	93
Ethical Considerations	95
Global Perspectives	96
Chapter Summary	98
The Road Ahead	99
Your Feedback Matters	109
About the Author	111

UNDERSTANDING THE GUT-BRAIN CONNECTION

Imagine your gut as a bustling metropolis, teeming with microbes that influence your mood, thoughts, and decisions. This isn't science fiction; it's the reality of the gut-brain connection. This complex communication network, also known as the gut-brain axis, links your central nervous system to your enteric nervous system. The connection is so powerful that some scientists call this system the "second brain."

The vagus nerve is at the heart of this connection, a two-way superhighway that transmits signals between the brain and digestive system. This nerve plays a crucial role in monitoring and integrating gut functions. It is a key player in the physical manifestations of our emotions.

But the communication isn't just neural. It's chemical too. The gut is a major site for producing neurotransmitters, such as serotonin, which plays an important role in regulating mood. This means that the state of your gut can directly influence your emotional well-being.

The gut microbiome, the vast community of microorganisms in our digestive system, also plays a pivotal role in this communication network. These microbes can produce substances that affect the brain, influence our immune system, and even modulate our stress response. Changes in the composition of the gut microbiota have been linked to a variety of neurological and psychiatric disorders, highlighting the importance of maintaining a healthy gut for mental well-being.

Understanding the gut-brain axis opens new avenues for treating mental and physical health issues. It's a fascinating reminder of how interconnected our bodies are and how much our gut feelings matter.

As we delve deeper into the mysteries of the gut-brain connection, we'll embark on a journey that challenges our understanding of the mind-body relationship. It promises not only to revolutionize our approach to health and disease but also to illuminate the intricate ways in which our bodies speak to us if only we learn to listen.

HISTORICAL PERSPECTIVES

The gut-brain connection is not a concept that began in the modern era. Its roots stretch far back into history, weaving through centuries of medical theories and practices. The ancient Greeks, for instance, were proponents of the idea that the gut's health was intrinsically linked to the well-being of the mind and body. Hippocrates, often hailed as the father of medicine, famously said, "*All disease begins in the gut*". This statement, though simplistic by today's standards, hinted at an understanding that the digestive system plays a crucial role in overall health, a notion that has evolved and expanded with time.

Fast-forward to the 19th and early 20th centuries, when the scientific community began to take a more detailed interest in the mechanics of digestion and the nervous system. Researchers started to uncover the complex ways in which the gut and the brain communicate through direct neural connections, hormones, and the immune system. Yet, despite these advances, the gut-brain axis remained a peripheral area of study, overshadowed by other medical discoveries of the time.

In the late 20th and early 21st centuries, the gut-brain connection began to emerge as a central area of interest, thanks in part to the advent of sophisticated research techniques. Scientists were able to delve deeper into the microbiome—the vast ecosystem of bacteria, viruses, and fungi that reside in the gut—and its potential impact on mental health, cognitive function, and neurological diseases.

I remember my grandmother often saying, *"Listen to your gut"*. As a child, I took her advice literally, thinking only of the rumblings of hunger or the discomfort of overeating. Much later, immersed in the complexities of gut-brain research, I appreciated the depth of her wisdom. Our ancestors might not have had the scientific tools we possess today. Still, they recognized the importance of the gut for overall well-being, a testament to the enduring nature of this connection through the ages.

Today, we stand on the brink of a new frontier in understanding the gut-brain axis. Each study reveals more about how this intricate relationship influences our health, emotions, and even our decisions. The historical journey of the gut-brain connection, from ancient wisdom to cutting-edge science, is a powerful reminder of the complexity of the human body and the interconnectedness of our physical and mental health. As we delve further into this fascinating topic, we honor the insights of the past while forging new paths in the quest for knowledge.

WHY IT MATTERS

Imagine, for a moment, that your body is a finely tuned orchestra. Each organ and system plays its part, contributing to the symphony that is your daily life. Now, consider the gut and the brain as two principal players in this orchestra. Traditionally, we've thought of them as entirely separate, each playing their own music, so to speak. But what if I told you they're performing a duet? This is the essence of the gut-brain connection, a fascinating dialogue between your digestive and central nervous systems.

Why does this matter? Well, this connection suggests that our mental and gut health are more intertwined than we ever imagined. Have you ever felt "butterflies" in your stomach before a big presentation? Have you experienced a "gut-wrenching" sensation during moments of stress? These are not just metaphors. They are real, physical reactions that occur due to the gut-brain connection.

But it goes deeper than just feelings. Research is now showing that the state of our gut can influence our mood, our mental health, and even our susceptibility to conditions like anxiety and depression. Conversely, our brain can affect the health and function of our gut. This two-way street is not just a scientific curiosity; it's a vital aspect of our health that we can no longer afford to ignore.

Understanding the gut-brain connection encourages us to look at our health holistically, recognizing that what we eat, how we feel, and how we live are all interconnected. It's a call to pay attention to our gut health, not just for the sake of our digestion but for our overall well-being.

Moreover, this connection highlights the importance of diet, stress management, and lifestyle choices in maintaining health. It's not just about avoiding illness; it's about fostering a state of wellness that encompasses both mind and body. By nurturing our gut-brain connection through healthy habits, we can enhance our resilience, mood, and overall quality of life.

So, why does the gut-brain connection matter? Because it's a fundamental part of who we are. It reminds us that every player in the complex orchestra of our body is connected, and by understanding these connections, we can live healthier, happier lives.

This journey into the gut-brain connection is not just about science; it's about discovering a more integrated approach to our health that honors the intricate symphony within us.

KEY CONCEPTS AND TERMS

Before we explore the gut-brain connection further, let's familiarize ourselves with some key concepts and terms that will frequently pop up throughout our journey. Understanding these will enhance our comprehension and allow us to appreciate the intricate dance between our gut and brain even more.

Gut-Brain Axis

First up is the gut-brain axis. This term refers to the complex communication network linking the gastrointestinal tract and the central nervous system. It's a bi-directional highway, with traffic flowing in both directions. Messages sent from the gut to the brain can influence our mood, stress levels, and even decision-making processes, while the brain can affect gut functions, impacting digestion, appetite, and more.

Microbiota

Next, let's talk about microbiota. This refers to the vast

community of microorganisms living in our digestive system. These tiny inhabitants play a massive role in our health, affecting everything from nutrient absorption to immune system function. The composition of your microbiota is as unique as a fingerprint. It's influenced by factors like diet, lifestyle, and even how you were born.

Neurotransmitters

Neurotransmitters are another key player. These chemical messengers are crucial for brain function, facilitating communication between neurons. Interestingly, many neurotransmitters, such as serotonin and dopamine, are also found in the gut, where they help regulate gut movements and influence gut-brain communication.

Inflammation

The term inflammation often appears in discussions about the gut-brain connection. While it's a natural immune response, chronic inflammation in the gut can lead to a host of problems, including mood disorders like depression and anxiety. This ties back to the gut-brain axis, as the health of our gut can directly impact our brain's well-being.

Probiotics and Prebiotics

Lastly, probiotics and prebiotics are worth noting. Probiotics are live bacteria and yeasts that are good for our health, especially our digestive system. Prebiotics, on the other hand, are types of dietary fiber that feed the beneficial bacteria in our gut. Both play a role in maintaining a healthy gut microbiota, which, as we've learned, is crucial for a healthy gut-brain connection.

UNDERSTANDING THE GUT-BRAIN CONNECTION

With these concepts and terms in our toolkit, we're better equipped to dive deeper into the fascinating world of the gut-brain connection. This journey promises to shed light on our gut health's profound impact on our overall well-being. So, let's continue, keeping these key concepts in mind as we unravel the mysteries of the gut-brain axis.

WHAT TO EXPECT FROM THIS BOOK

This book is designed to unravel the complex and important relationship between our gut and brain. So, what exactly can you expect as we delve deeper into this intriguing subject?

Firstly, we'll start with the basics, breaking down the science behind the gut-brain axis in a way that's both accessible and engaging. You don't need a PhD to follow along. We're talking clear explanations, relatable examples, and real-life applications. Whether you're a curious newcomer or someone with a bit of background knowledge, there's something here for you.

Why should you care? Well, that's a question we'll tackle head-on. The implications of the gut-brain connection touch on everything from mental health to chronic disease, diet, and beyond. Understanding this relationship can open doors to new ways of managing our well-being, making informed choices about our diet, and even improving our mental health.

Throughout this book, expect a blend of research, expert insights, and real-world stories that bring the gut-brain connection to life. We'll explore how this knowledge is applied in medicine, psychology, and everyday life, offering practical tips and strategies.

So, whether you're looking to improve your health, understand the science, or satisfy your curiosity, you're in the right place. Let's embark on this journey together, exploring the fascinating world of the gut-brain connection.

HOW TO USE THIS BOOK

This book is designed to be your map, your compass, and sometimes, your flashlight shining a light on the intricate pathways that link your gut to your brain. How you navigate through this book can significantly enhance your understanding and application of the knowledge within. So, let's talk about how to make the most of this journey.

First and foremost, approach this book with curiosity. Each section is crafted to build upon the last, starting with a broad overview and funneling into specific insights and actionable advice. Whether you're a healthcare professional, a student, or simply someone interested in the marvels of human biology, there's something here for you.

Science constantly evolves; what we know today might be the tip of the iceberg. This book sets the stage for why the gut-brain connection matters, not just for academic interest but for its implications on our health, well-being, and even behavior.

As you read the chapters, take notes. Jot down concepts that stand out to you, questions that arise, or even personal reflections on how the information resonates with your own experiences. These notes can become a personalized guide, helping you connect the dots in ways that are most meaningful to you.

Don't feel compelled to read from cover to cover in one go. While the book is structured to build your understanding in a logical sequence, it's also designed to allow you to jump to sections that particularly interest you. Feel free to skip ahead if you're drawn to the practical aspects, such as how to nurture your gut-brain connection through diet, lifestyle, or mindfulness. You can always circle back to fill in the gaps.

Finally, engage with the content. Reflect on how the information applies to your life. Experiment with the suggestions provided, whether it's tweaking your diet, trying new stress-reduction techniques, or simply observing how your gut feelings guide your decisions. This book is not just about acquiring knowledge; it's about translating it into actions that can improve your health and happiness.

Remember, this journey is personal. Your experiences, insights, and outcomes may differ from others, and that's perfectly okay. The goal is not just to learn about the gut-brain connection but to understand how it influences you and how you can harness its power to enhance your well-being.

So, take a deep breath, open your mind, and let's begin this fascinating exploration together. Welcome to the journey of understanding the gut-brain connection.

CHAPTER SUMMARY

- The gut-brain connection is a complex communication network linking the brain and gut. It reveals a complex relationship between our digestive system and brain that influences mood, health, and decisions.
- The vagus nerve is a crucial component of this connection. It transmits signals between the brain and the digestive system, affecting emotions and physical responses.
- The gut produces neurotransmitters like serotonin, which significantly influences mood and emotional well-being. Ninety percent of the body's serotonin is produced in the digestive tract.

- The gut microbiome consists of microorganisms in the digestive system. It plays a vital role in affecting the brain, immune system, and stress response. Its composition is linked to various neurological and psychiatric disorders.
- Understanding the gut-brain axis suggests that maintaining gut health through diet and lifestyle changes can impact mood, cognitive function, and overall health.
- Historical perspectives show that the exploration of the gut-brain connection dates back to ancient times, with modern scientific advancements providing deeper insights into its significance.
- The gut-brain connection matters because it highlights the interconnection between mental and physical health, suggesting that gut health can influence mental health and vice versa.
- Key concepts related to the gut-brain connection include the gut-brain axis, microbiota, neurotransmitters, inflammation, probiotics, and prebiotics, essential for understanding the relationship between gut health and overall well-being.

CHAPTER 1
THE SCIENCE OF THE GUT-BRAIN CONNECTION

The gut-brain connection influences our health, mood, and decisions in a fundamental way. It's a story of how two seemingly distinct body parts are intricately linked. It begins with understanding the key players: the gut, the brain, and the vast network that connects them.

At the heart of this connection is the enteric nervous system (ENS), often dubbed the "second brain." Nestled within the walls of our gut, the ENS consists of over 100 million nerve cells lining our gastrointestinal tract from the esophagus to the rectum. Its primary role is to control digestion, from the breaking down of food to the absorption of nutrients and the expulsion of waste. But its influence stretches far beyond, directly communicating with the brain.

This communication happens via multiple mechanisms, including the vagus nerve, one of the longest nerves in the body. Then there's the microbiome, a vast ecosystem of bacteria residing in our gut, which plays a crucial role in this dialogue. These microbes help digest our food and produce substances that can affect our brain, influencing our emotions, how we perceive pain, and even our behaviors.

I remember a time when I was preparing for an important presentation. My nerves were high, and my stomach felt like it was in knots. It was a visceral reminder of how stress can manifest physically in our gut, affecting digestion and comfort. This experience, though seemingly small, shows the important impact of the gut-brain connection on our daily lives, influencing not just our physical health but our mental well-being too.

As we delve deeper into the science of the gut-brain connection, we'll explore the mechanisms of this communication, the role of the microbiome, and the implications for health and disease. This journey promises to reshape our understanding of the human body, offering new pathways for healing and wellness. So, let's continue this exploration together, unraveling the mysteries of the gut-brain connection and its profound impact on our lives.

NEUROTRANSMITTERS AND HORMONES

We uncover the fascinating dialogue between our gut and brain first through the intricate world of neurotransmitters and hormones. This conversation, primarily chemical in nature, is pivotal for our overall well-being. Let's break it down, shall we?

Neurotransmitters, the brain's chemical messengers, play a crucial role in this communication. Serotonin, often dubbed the "feel-good" neurotransmitter, is a prime example. Surprisingly, about 90% of our body's serotonin is produced in the gut. This fact alone demonstrates the gut's significant influence on our mood and emotional health. Then there's gamma-aminobutyric acid, another neurotransmitter involved in regulating anxiety. Its production, too, is influenced by gut bacteria, highlighting how our microbiome can be a powerful ally in managing stress.

Hormones, on the other hand, are like the body's long-distance messengers. They travel through the bloodstream, affecting various processes. Cortisol, the stress hormone, is one such messenger. Its levels can be influenced by both the brain's perception of stress and the gut's response to it. Depending on the state of our gut health, this interplay can either ramp up our stress response or help dial it down.

Understanding the roles of neurotransmitters and hormones in the gut-brain connection allows us to discover new ways to enhance our mental and physical health. It becomes not just about what we eat, but how what we eat influences our feelings, thoughts, and overall well-being.

The gut-brain axis, with its complex web of chemical signals, offers a fascinating glimpse into the holistic nature of health. By nurturing our gut, we're not just taking care of our digestive health; we're taking a step towards a happier, more balanced mind.

THE ROLE OF THE MICROBIOME

Dive into the bustling world of your gut, and you'll find a complex ecosystem that's more influential than you might have imagined. This ecosystem, known as the microbiome, is a community of trillions of bacteria, viruses, fungi, and other microorganisms living in your digestive system. But it's not just a crowded space; it's a dynamic one that plays a pivotal role in your health, particularly in how your brain functions. Let's explore how this fascinating world within us impacts our brain and overall well-being.

First, it's essential to understand that the microbiome is not a static entity. It changes based on diet, lifestyle, age, and even the environment. This means that the choices you make every day, from what you eat to how much you sleep, can influence the composition of your gut flora. And why does this matter? The state of your microbiome can affect everything from your mood to your susceptibility to diseases.

The connection between the gut and the brain is a two-way street. Signals from the brain can influence gut activity. Conversely, the gut can send messages to the brain. This communication happens through various pathways, including the nervous system, immune system, and hormones. But the microbiome plays a starring role in this complex communication network.

One of the microbiome's most fascinating aspects is its effect on mental health. Research has shown that certain bacteria in the gut can produce neurotransmitters, such as serotonin and dopamine, which are critical for mood regulation. This means that the composition of your microbiome could directly impact your feelings of happiness and anxiety.

Moreover, the gut microbiome can affect the body's stress response. A healthy, balanced microbiome may moderate the body's reaction to stress, potentially reducing the risk of stress-related disorders. On the flip side, an imbalanced microbiome, known as dysbiosis, can exacerbate the body's stress response, potentially leading to a higher risk of anxiety and depression.

The implications of the gut-brain connection extend beyond mental health. There's growing evidence to suggest that the microbiome may play a role in neurodegenerative diseases, such as Alzheimer's and Parkinson's disease. While research is still in its early stages, it's a promising area that could open up new approaches for prevention and treatment.

In conclusion, the microbiome is critical in the gut-brain connection, influencing our mental health, stress response, and potentially even the risk of neurodegenerative diseases.

Taking care of your gut is not just about avoiding stomach aches or digestive issues; it's also about nurturing your mental and emotional well-being. As we continue to unravel the mysteries of the gut-brain connection, we are learning that the path to a happier, healthier life might just start with our gut. By taking steps to support a healthy microbiome, we're not just taking care of our gut; we're taking care of our brain, too.

RESEARCH AND EVIDENCE

The connection between our gut and brain is not just a fascinating topic for casual conversation; it's a rapidly evolving field backed by a growing body of research. The evidence we're about to explore sheds light on how deeply interconnected our digestive system and brain are and the implications of this relationship for our health and well-being.

Let's start with a groundbreaking study that turned heads and opened minds. Researchers have already discovered that the gut microbiome, that is, the trillions of bacteria residing in our digestive tract, communicates directly with the brain through the gut-brain axis. This communication happens via various pathways, including the vagus nerve. It's like a two-way street, with traffic flowing in both directions, carrying messages that affect mood, stress levels, and even decision-making.

Further studies have delved into the impact of the gut microbiome on neurodevelopmental disorders, such as autism spectrum disorder (ASD). Researchers have found distinct differences in the gut bacteria of individuals with ASD compared to those without, pointing towards the gut-brain connection as a potential area for therapeutic intervention.

The evidence doesn't stop there. Clinical trials have begun to explore the use of probiotics as a treatment for depression and anxiety, with some promising results. These studies suggest that altering the gut microbiome's composition may alleviate symptoms of mental health disorders.

In a particularly intriguing study, scientists transplanted the gut microbiota from depressed humans into mice, which then began to exhibit depressive-like behaviors. This experiment further shows the potential of the gut microbiome to influence brain function and behavior.

As we sift through the evidence provided by such studies, it becomes clear that the gut-brain connection is more than just a scientific curiosity. It's a vital aspect of our health that could unlock new frontiers in the treatment of mental health disorders, among other conditions. The research is still in its early stages, but the possibilities are exciting and vast.

CHALLENGES AND LIMITATIONS

Diving into the science of the gut-brain connection opens up a world of fascinating insights and potential breakthroughs in understanding human health. However, as with any field of scientific inquiry, there are challenges and limitations that must be acknowledged. These hurdles shape the current state of research and guide future investigations.

One of the primary challenges in studying the gut-brain connection is the complexity of the systems involved. The human gut microbiome is a vast and diverse ecosystem comprising hundreds of species of bacteria, each with its role in health and disease. Similarly, the brain is one of the most complex organs in the body, responsible for processing billions of bits of information every second. Unraveling the interactions between these two systems is no small feat. Researchers must navigate this complexity, often relying on animal models or in vitro studies that may only partially replicate human physiology.

Another hurdle is the variability among individuals. Each person's microbiome is as unique as their fingerprint, influenced by factors such as diet, lifestyle, and genetics. This variability can make it challenging to draw broad conclusions from research findings. What works for one person in terms of diet or probiotic supplementation may have a different effect on someone else, complicating the development of universal guidelines for improving gut-brain health.

The field also faces methodological limitations. Many studies on the gut-brain axis are observational, which can identify correlations but not prove causation. While these studies are valuable for generating hypotheses, more rigorous, controlled trials are needed to establish transparent cause-and-effect relationships. However, such trials are expensive, time-consuming, and fraught with ethical considerations, especially when involving interventions that may affect mental health.

Despite these challenges, the pursuit of understanding the gut-brain connection is more than a scientific endeavor; it's a journey toward unlocking new ways to improve human health. Researchers are continually developing more sophisticated tools and methods to study this complex relationship, from advanced imaging techniques to novel computational models that can analyze vast datasets.

As we navigate these challenges and limitations, it's crucial to approach findings with a critical eye and a healthy dose of skepticism. The science of the gut-brain connection is still in its infancy, and while the potential is enormous, there is much we still need to learn. By acknowledging these hurdles, we can better appreciate the progress made so far and the journey ahead.

CHAPTER SUMMARY

- The gut-brain connection is a complex, bidirectional communication system that influences health, mood, and decisions. It involves the gut, brain, and enteric nervous system (ENS).
- The ENS controls digestion and communicates directly with the brain through pathways like the vagus nerve and the microbiome, affecting emotions and behaviors.
- Stress and anxiety can physically manifest in the gut, affecting digestion and comfort. This highlights the gut-brain connection's impact on daily life and mental well-being.
- Neurotransmitters and hormones, such as serotonin and GABA, are significantly influenced by gut bacteria, affecting mood and stress levels.
- The microbiome, a dynamic ecosystem within the gut, plays a crucial role in mental health, stress response, and potentially neurodegenerative diseases influenced by diet and lifestyle.
- Research supports the gut-brain connection, showing direct communication through the gut-brain axis and the influence of gut bacteria on neurotransmitters and mental health. Probiotics show promise in treating depression and anxiety.
- Challenges in studying the gut-brain connection include the complexity of the systems, individual variability, and methodological limitations, emphasizing the need for cautious interpretation of findings and further research.

CHAPTER 2
DIET AND THE GUT-BRAIN CONNECTION

Imagine your gut as a bustling city with trillions of residents, including bacteria, viruses, and fungi. This city's health directly impacts your own, influencing everything from your mood to your susceptibility to illness. Now, consider your diet as the policy decisions that shape this city. What you eat can support a thriving metropolis or lead to a neglected town.

Foods rich in fiber, such as fruits, vegetables, and whole grains, act like the city's infrastructure projects, supporting the growth of beneficial bacteria. These good bacteria are crucial. They help digest food, produce vitamins, and protect against pathogens. In essence, a diet high in fiber is like investing in roads, parks, and schools for our gut city, fostering a community where health can flourish.

Conversely, a diet high in processed foods and sugars is akin to allowing pollution to overrun our city. Such foods can promote the growth of harmful bacteria and yeasts, leading to a disrupted gut environment. This disruption can manifest in various ways, from minor discomforts like bloating and gas to more severe conditions like irritable bowel syndrome and inflammatory bowel disease.

But it's not just about what we eat; it's also about how we eat. The modern lifestyle often promotes eating quickly, under stress, or on the go. This way of eating can hinder the digestive process and the absorption of nutrients, further impacting gut health. Taking the time to eat mindfully in a relaxed setting can enhance our gut's ability to process and benefit from the nutrients in our food.

The impact of diet on gut health is undeniable. By choosing foods that nourish our gut bacteria, we're not just feeding ourselves; we're nurturing the complex ecosystem within us that plays a crucial role in our overall health. It's a reminder that in the quest for well-being, the journey starts not with a single step but with a single bite.

FOODS TO FAVOR

When we talk about nourishing our bodies, we're not just fueling up like cars at a gas station. It's more intricate, more intimate. What we eat doesn't just power us through the day; it communicates with our gut and, in turn, our brain. This dialogue between our gut and brain is a fascinating conversation. So, let's dive into the foods that can make this conversation as positive and beneficial as possible.

Fiber-Rich Foods

First up, let's talk about fiber. It's not the most glamorous of nutrients, but it's a superstar when it comes to gut health. Foods rich in fiber, like fruits, vegetables, legumes, and whole grains, are like the life of the party in your gut. They feed the good bacteria, helping them thrive and multiply. This is crucial because a happy, healthy gut microbiome is linked to a happier, healthier brain. Think of fiber as the facilitator of a good chat between your gut and brain, keeping the lines of communication open and positive.

Fermented Foods

Next, we must recognize the importance of fermented foods. These foods have been through a process that allows natural bacteria to ferment the sugar and starch, creating lactic acid. This process not only preserves these foods but also creates beneficial enzymes, b-vitamins, Omega-3 fatty acids, and various strains of probiotics. Yogurt, kefir, sauerkraut, kimchi, and kombucha are all excellent examples. Including these in your diet can help increase the diversity of your gut flora, which, in turn, can enhance your gut-brain communication.

Prebiotics

Prebiotic foods are another cornerstone of a gut-healthy diet. Prebiotics feed the beneficial bacteria in our gut, helping to stimulate their growth and activity. Prebiotic-rich foods include garlic, onions, leeks, asparagus, bananas, and whole grains. By nourishing the beneficial bacteria in our gut, prebiotics help to maintain a balanced ecosystem, which is essential for both digestive health and mental well-being. They also provide many vitamins and minerals crucial for brain function.

Omega-3 Fatty Acids

Omega-3 fatty acids are another key player. Found in fatty fish like salmon, mackerel, and sardines, as well as in flaxseeds, chia seeds, and walnuts, Omega-3s are essential for brain health. They help build cell membranes in the brain and have anti-inflammatory properties. By reducing inflammation, they can potentially reduce symptoms of depression and anxiety.

Antioxidants

Antioxidants also deserve a shoutout. These compounds, found in colorful fruits and vegetables, nuts, seeds, and even dark chocolate, protect your body from oxidative stress, which can damage cells. By fighting this stress, antioxidants can help maintain the integrity of the gut lining, ensuring that the gut-brain communication line remains strong and clear.

Water

Lastly, let's not forget about hydration. Water might not be a 'food,' per se, but it's essential for every cell in your body to function correctly, including those in your gut and brain. Staying hydrated helps ensure that nutrients are transported efficiently, toxins are flushed out, and the tissues in your gut and brain stay healthy.

Incorporating these foods into your diet isn't just about avoiding illness or trying to 'fix' something; it's about nurturing a positive, supportive dialogue between your gut and brain. It's about creating a foundation for mental and physical health that supports you in living your best life. So, the next time you eat, think about what messages you're sending inside. It's not just food; it's a conversation.

FOODS TO AVOID

We've explored the foods that nourish and support the intricate relationship between your gut and brain. Now, let's pivot to the other side of the coin—foods that might be doing more harm than good. It's a journey of discovery, one that even took me by surprise as I delved deeper into the research and reflected on my own eating habits.

Processed Foods

First up, let's talk about processed foods. These items are packed with additives, preservatives, and artificial ingredients far removed from their natural state. Think about those microwave meals, canned goods with long shelf lives, and snacks that crunch a little too perfectly. They're convenient, sure, but they're also associated with inflammation and disruptions in the gut microbiome, which can send ripple effects to our brain, impacting mood and cognitive function.

Sugar

Then, there's sugar. Oh, sugar. It's everywhere, from bread to sauces, hiding in places you wouldn't expect. While I've always had a bit of a sweet tooth, learning about how high sugar intake can lead to an imbalance in gut bacteria and potentially contribute to anxiety and depression was a wake-up call. It's not about cutting it out entirely—life's too short not to enjoy a slice of cake at a party—but about being mindful of the hidden sugars in our daily diet.

Artificial Sweeteners

Artificial sweeteners are another culprit. To dodge the calories from sugar, many turn to these synthetic substitutes. However, studies suggest they may negatively affect the gut microbiome and insulin sensitivity. It's a classic case of solving one problem but potentially creating another.

Trans Fats

Trans fats, found in some fried foods, baked goods, and processed snacks, are also on the list. These fats are notorious for their role in heart disease but are also implicated in causing inflammation and harming gut health. Remembering the times I'd indulge in a late-night fast-food run, it's clear that the temporary comfort was not worth the long-term impact on my well-being.

Alcohol

Lastly, let's not forget about alcohol. In moderation, it can be part of a balanced lifestyle. Still, excessive consumption is a known antagonist to gut health, leading to imbalances that affect both physical and mental health. Reflecting on my own experiences, cutting back on alcohol was a personal decision that really improved my overall mood and energy levels.

This section is not about fear or avoiding certain foods forever. It's about awareness and making informed choices that support our gut-brain connection, leading to a happier, healthier life. As we continue this journey together, remember that small changes can make a big difference.

PROBIOTICS AND PREBIOTICS

Though often mentioned in the same breath, probiotics and prebiotics perform distinct roles in our digestive system and can influence our mental and physical health. Let's explore their impact on gut health in more detail.

Probiotics are the live bacteria and yeasts that are good for our digestive system. They're often called "good" or "helpful" bacteria because they help keep our gut healthy. Found in various foods and supplements, these microorganisms can enhance the gut microbiota, which is crucial for our overall health. By consuming probiotics, we add beneficial players to this microbial community, promoting a balance supporting gut and brain health.

Prebiotics, on the other hand, are types of dietary fiber that feed the friendly bacteria in our gut. Think of them as the fuel that helps the good bacteria grow and flourish. Various fruits, vegetables, and whole grains contain these nondigestible food components. By nourishing the beneficial bacteria, prebiotics help enhance digestion and absorption of nutrients and significantly impact the production of neurotransmitters and hormones that regulate mood and cognitive functions.

The synergy between probiotics and prebiotics is crucial for maintaining a healthy gut-brain axis. Recent research suggests that a healthy gut microbiota can positively affect communication between the emotional and cognitive centers of the brain and intestinal functions. For instance, certain strains of probiotics have been shown to produce neurotransmitters like serotonin and dopamine, playing a pivotal role in regulating mood and emotions.

Incorporating various probiotic and prebiotic-rich foods into your diet can be a simple yet effective way to support this connection. As mentioned earlier, yogurt, kefir, sauerkraut, and miso are excellent sources of probiotics. Bananas, onions, garlic, and asparagus are great for prebiotic intake. However, it's important to remember that balance is vital. Just as a diverse diet supports a diverse microbiome, incorporating a wide range of probiotic and prebiotic foods can help ensure a healthy gut-brain axis.

DIETARY PLANS AND RECOMMENDATIONS

Navigating the vast sea of dietary advice can feel overwhelming, especially when trying to enhance your gut-brain connection. But fear not! The key is to embrace a balanced, diverse diet rich in whole foods. This approach not only supports your gut microbiome but also your overall mental and physical health. Let's dive into some actionable recommendations to help you craft a diet that fosters a happy gut and brain.

Strive For Variety

First off, variety is your best friend. Incorporating a wide range of fruits, vegetables, whole grains, lean proteins, and healthy fats ensures you get a broad spectrum of nutrients and prebiotics essential for a thriving microbiome. Think colorful plates filled with dark leafy greens, bright berries, and vibrant vegetables. These are pleasing to the eye and packed with vitamins, minerals, and fibers that support gut health.

Add Fiber

Fiber is a superstar when it comes to feeding the good bacteria in your gut. Aim for a mix of soluble and insoluble fiber from sources like oats, apples, carrots, beans, and flaxseeds. These foods help keep things moving in your digestive system and can prevent that sluggish feeling that comes from a less-than-ideal diet.

Incorporate Probiotics

Probiotics are another cornerstone of gut health, introducing beneficial bacteria to your digestive system. Fermented foods are excellent sources of probiotics. A high-quality probiotic supplement can also do the trick if you're not a fan of these flavors. Just be sure to check with a healthcare professional before starting any new supplement regimen.

Remember to Hydrate

Now, let's talk hydration. Remember that water plays a crucial role in digestion and absorption, helping to break down food and transport nutrients to your cells. Aim to drink plenty of water throughout the day. Foods like cucumbers, watermelon, and oranges can also contribute to your daily fluid intake.

Limited Processed Foods, Sugar and Unhealthy Fats

While focusing on what to add to your diet, it's equally important to consider what to limit. Processed foods, high in sugar and unhealthy fats, can disrupt your gut microbiome and lead to inflammation, affecting both your gut and brain health. Try to minimize these foods, opting for whole, nutrient-dense options instead.

Gradual Adjustments

Lastly, remember that change doesn't happen overnight.

Gradually incorporating these dietary adjustments allows your body to adapt and makes it easier to stick to these healthier habits in the long run. Listen to your body, and don't hesitate to consult a nutritionist or dietitian to tailor these recommendations to your needs and goals.

By embracing these dietary plans and recommendations, you're not just feeding your body; you're nourishing your brain and fostering a stronger, more resilient gut-brain connection. Here's to a happier, healthier you!

CASE STUDIES

Diet has the power to transform the gut-brain connection. The stories of individuals who have navigated the journey from discomfort and imbalance to wellness and vitality are not just inspiring; they demonstrate how our dietary choices impact our mental and physical health. Let's delve into a few of these remarkable stories, shedding light on the benefits of nurturing our gut-brain axis with thoughtful nutrition.

First, meet Alex. Alex's life was once ruled by anxiety and digestive discomfort, a duo that kept him in a constant state of unease. Traditional medications provided temporary relief but didn't address the root of his issues. The turning point came when he decided to overhaul his diet, focusing on whole foods, probiotics, and prebiotics while reducing the amount of packaged and processed foods he ate. Within weeks, Alex noticed a significant decrease in his anxiety levels and a dramatic improvement in his digestive health. This change wasn't just physical but deeply emotional, empowering Alex to regain control over his life.

Then there's Priya, who struggled with irritable bowel

syndrome (IBS) and depression for years. The link between her gut health and mental state was a puzzle she couldn't solve until she was introduced to the concept of the gut-brain connection. By adopting a diet rich in anti-inflammatory foods and cutting out gluten and dairy, Priya began to see improvements in her symptoms. Her journey was not without challenges, but her persistence paid off, leading to a noticeable reduction in her IBS flare-ups and a more positive outlook on life.

Lastly, consider the story of Jordan, who suffered from chronic fatigue and brain fog, making it difficult to concentrate and stay productive throughout the day. The breakthrough came when Jordan decided to experiment with a ketogenic diet, aiming to stabilize blood sugar levels and reduce inflammation. The results were nothing short of transformative. Not only did Jordan's energy levels soar, but the mental clarity he experienced allowed him to enjoy activities he had previously given up on.

These stories are more than just individual successes; they are a beacon of hope for anyone looking to improve their health through dietary changes. They reveal the importance of listening to our bodies and being open to adjusting our eating habits for the sake of our well-being.

While each person's path to health is unique, the underlying message is clear: the food we eat plays a crucial role in the intricate dance between our gut and brain. We can embark on a healthier, happier life by embracing this connection and making more informed dietary choices.

CHAPTER SUMMARY

- Diet plays a crucial role in gut health, affecting mood and disease susceptibility.

- High-fiber foods support beneficial gut bacteria, while processed foods and sugars can disrupt the gut environment and lead to health issues.
- Mindful eating in a relaxed setting enhances nutrient absorption and overall gut health.
- Fiber-rich foods, fermented foods, Omega-3 fatty acids, antioxidants, and staying hydrated are recommended for a healthy gut-brain dialogue.
- To prevent negative impacts on gut health, processed foods, high sugar intake, artificial sweeteners, trans fats, and excessive alcohol should be minimized or avoided.
- Probiotics and prebiotics play distinct roles in digestive health, influencing mental and physical well-being through the gut-brain axis.
- Embracing a balanced diet rich in whole foods, variety, and specific gut-supportive nutrients is vital to fostering a healthy gut-brain connection.

CHAPTER 3
STRESS, EMOTIONS, AND THE GUT

When we talk about stress, it's not just a feeling. Stress is a complex, full-body response that deeply affects our gut. Your brain and gut are in constant conversation, and stress is like static interference disrupting their dialogue. This interference can lead to a range of gut issues, from minor discomfort to more serious conditions.

The stress response, often called 'fight or flight,' is our body's ancient reaction to perceived threats. It's designed to protect us by preparing our bodies to either face the danger or run away from it. This response involves a cascade of hormones, including cortisol and adrenaline, which have immediate and powerful effects on our body. One of these effects is the redirection of blood flow away from the gut, prioritizing muscles and other organs essential for quick action.

But here's the kicker: our modern lives rarely require us to actually fight or flee. Yet, our bodies react to modern stressors - deadlines, traffic, personal conflicts - with the same intensity as they would to a life-threatening situation. This means our gut frequently misses out on the blood flow, oxygen, and nutrients it needs for proper digestion and function.

Stress can also alter the gut's permeability, sometimes called 'leaky gut,' allowing bacteria and toxins to pass into the bloodstream. This can trigger inflammation and changes in the gut microbiome. When stress disrupts the microbiome, it can really affect our health.

Imagine this: Sarah, a 35-year-old project manager, is in the middle of a high-stakes project. Deadlines are looming, the pressure is mounting, and her stomach is in knots. She notices that her digestion is off, she's experiencing bloating, and her usual healthy appetite has dwindled. This isn't a coincidence. Sarah's stress is not just affecting her mind; it's also taking a toll on her gut health.

Many of us have experienced similar situations where stress leads to noticeable changes in our digestive system. The reason? Our gut is incredibly sensitive to emotions and stress through the gut-brain axis. When we're stressed, our brain sends signals to our gut, which can lead to various gastrointestinal symptoms.

But it's not all doom and gloom. Understanding the connection between stress and the gut allows us to focus on practices that help manage stress and improve gut health. Simple practices like mindfulness, deep breathing exercises, and regular physical activity can help mitigate the stress response and its effects on the gut. Paying attention to our diet and ensuring we consume foods that support gut health can also make a big difference.

Managing stress is not just about feeling better mentally; it's about taking care of our entire body, including our gut.

MANAGING STRESS FOR GUT HEALTH

Stress seems like an unwelcome guest that never entirely leaves in the hustle and bustle of our daily lives. It's no secret that stress can wreak havoc on our mental health, and we discovered earlier that it can also significantly impact our gut health. But here's the good news: just as stress can impact our gut, improving gut health can positively influence our emotional well-being and ability to handle stress.

Let's look at some practical steps you can take to reduce stress and take better care of your gut.

Mindfulness and Meditation

First off, mindfulness and meditation have shown promising results. These practices help calm the mind, reduce stress levels, and, in turn, can lead to a happier gut. It's like sending a peace treaty down your nervous system, letting your gut know it's safe to relax.

Exercise

Exercise is another powerful tool. But it's not just about getting fit or losing weight. Regular physical activity can help reduce stress levels. Whether it's a brisk walk, a yoga session, or a dance class, moving your body releases endorphins, the body's natural stress relievers. Plus, it's a great way to distract yourself from daily worries. We'll dive into this more in the next chapter.

Sleep

Now, let's talk about sleep. In our always-on world, sleep

often takes a backseat. However, quality sleep is a cornerstone of stress management and, by extension, gut health. Establishing a soothing bedtime routine and aiming for 7-9 hours of sleep can do wonders for your stress levels and gut. We'll explore the link between sleep and gut health in a future chapter.

Diet

Diet also plays a role in managing stress. A balanced diet rich in fruits, vegetables, whole grains, and lean proteins can help stabilize mood and reduce stress. On the other hand, high-sugar and high-fat foods can increase stress levels and inflammation, further aggravating gut issues.

Seeking Professional Help

Sometimes, the best course of action is to seek help from a professional. Cognitive-behavioral therapy and other therapeutic approaches can be incredibly effective in managing stress and improving gut health.

The Power of Connection

Lastly, don't underestimate the power of connection. Social support from friends, family, or support groups can provide a buffer against stress. Sharing your worries and joys with others can help reduce stress and its impact on your gut health.

Remember, managing stress is not about eliminating it altogether—that's impossible. Instead, it's about finding effective ways to cope with stress so it doesn't overwhelm you or your gut. By incorporating these strategies into your life, you're taking care of your mental health and nurturing your gut, strengthening that intricate connection between your brain and your gut.

MINDFULNESS AND MEDITATION

Mindfulness and meditation can be powerful tools in restoring harmony to our gut-brain axis.

Mindfulness is the practice of being present and fully engaged with whatever we're doing at the moment, free from distraction or judgment. It's about noticing the world around us and within us, acknowledging our thoughts and feelings without letting them overpower us. Meditation, often used alongside mindfulness, provides a structured approach to quieting the mind and finding peace. Together, they offer a sanctuary from the storm of stress and anxiety.

So, how exactly do mindfulness and meditation benefit our gut health? It all boils down to the stress response. By reducing stress and calming the mind, these practices can help mitigate the adverse effects of stress hormones on our gut. They encourage relaxation, which allows our digestive system to function more efficiently and reduces inflammation.

Moreover, mindfulness and meditation can enhance our emotional well-being, which is intrinsically linked to gut health. By fostering a sense of calm and reducing anxiety, mindfulness and meditation can help alleviate these physical symptoms and promote a healthier gut.

Incorporating mindfulness and meditation into your daily routine doesn't have to be daunting. It can be as simple as dedicating a few minutes daily to focus on your breath, practicing mindful eating, or engaging in guided meditation sessions. The key is consistency and patience. Like any skill, mindfulness and meditation take time to develop. Still, the benefits for your mind, body, and gut are well worth the effort.

Another way you can integrate mindfulness into your day is through mindful eating. Slow down and pay attention to what you're eating. This practice combines the knowledge we've gained on nutrition and mindfulness so far; it can help improve digestion and reduce stress levels. By taking the time to eat your meals without distractions, you can enjoy your food more and experience fewer digestive issues.

As we navigate the complexities of the gut-brain connection, it becomes clear that taking care of our mental health is just as important as maintaining our physical health. Mindfulness and meditation offer a bridge between the two, providing a holistic approach to wellness that nurtures our emotional well-being and gut health. So, next time you feel the weight of stress bearing down on you, remember that peace and balance are just a breath away.

THERAPEUTIC APPROACHES

When we dive into the realm of therapeutic approaches for managing the dance between stress, emotions, and our gut, we're exploring a treasure trove of strategies that can significantly enhance our well-being. It's a journey that takes us beyond conventional medicine, inviting us to consider holistic and integrative practices that honor the deep connection between our mind and body.

Cognitive-Behavioral Therapy

First, let's talk about cognitive-behavioral therapy (CBT). CBT is not just for the mind. It can be a powerful tool in understanding and changing the patterns of thought and behavior that influence our gut health. By addressing stress and anxiety, CBT helps mitigate their effects on our digestive system. It's like rewiring our brain to foster a healthier gut.

Hypnotherapy

Another fascinating approach is hypnotherapy. Yes, you read that right. Hypnotherapy isn't about stage tricks or mind control; it's a clinical practice that guides individuals into a deep state of relaxation, allowing them to tap into their subconscious to effect positive changes in their gut health. Studies have shown it to be particularly effective for conditions like irritable bowel syndrome.

The journey to managing stress, emotions, and gut health is multifaceted. It's about looking beyond the symptoms to the interconnectedness of our entire being. Whether through therapy, diet, exercise, or mindfulness, each step is towards a harmonious gut-brain connection. And remember, this journey is deeply personal. What works for one may not work for another. It's all about finding the right mix that resonates with your body and mind.

By understanding the intricate relationship between stress, emotions, and the gut, we can take proactive steps to manage stress and support our gut health. It's a journey of self-discovery, where small changes can improve our overall well-being.

CHAPTER SUMMARY

- Stress is a full-body response that significantly affects the gut. It disrupts the communication between the

brain and the gut and leads to various digestive issues.
- The stress response, or 'fight or flight,' redirects blood flow away from the gut, affecting digestion and nutrient absorption. It can also alter gut permeability, leading to a 'leaky gut.'
- Modern stressors trigger the same intense bodily reactions as life-threatening situations, affecting the gut's function and health due to reduced blood flow and nutrient supply.
- Stress can change the gut microbiome, impacting overall health, mood, and the immune system. However, managing stress through mindfulness, exercise, and diet can improve gut health.
- Emotional well-being is closely linked to gut health. Stress and negative emotions can disrupt gut function, while a healthy gut can enhance emotional resilience.
- Practical stress management techniques for gut health include mindfulness, meditation, regular exercise, quality sleep, a balanced diet, and social support.
- Mindfulness and meditation reduce stress and its harmful effects on the gut by promoting relaxation and improving digestive function and inflammation.
- Therapeutic approaches like cognitive-behavioral therapy and hypnotherapy can enhance the gut-brain connection and overall well-being.

CHAPTER 4
EXERCISE AND THE GUT-BRAIN AXIS

When we talk about the benefits of exercise, it's easy to think first of toned muscles, weight loss, and improved cardiovascular health. But there's another, less visible realm where the impact of regular exercise is just as meaningful: the gut-brain axis. Recent research has illuminated how exercise is pivotal in enhancing this connection, offering benefits beyond the gym.

First, exercise has been shown to promote a healthy balance of gut microbiota, which, as we learned, influences everything from digestion to immune function to mood regulation. Regular physical activity can increase the diversity of these microbiota, which is associated with better health outcomes. It's like a garden; the more variety you have, the more resilient it becomes.

Exercise also stimulates the production of short-chain fatty acids in the gut. These compounds have several beneficial effects, including strengthening the gut barrier, reducing inflammation, and providing energy to colon cells. This can lead to a healthier gut environment and, by extension, a more robust gut-brain communication.

Physical activity boosts the production of neurotrophic factors in the brain, such as brain-derived neurotrophic factor (BDNF). BDNF supports the survival of existing neurons and encourages the growth of new neurons and synapses. It's like fertilizer for the brain, enhancing brain plasticity, which can lead to improved cognitive function and a lower risk of mental health disorders.

Exercise also plays a significant role in managing stress, which can directly impact gut health. By reducing stress levels, exercise helps maintain a healthier gut environment, demonstrating how interconnected our physical activity and gut health are.

In essence, the benefits of physical activity extend far beyond what we can see. By engaging in regular exercise, we're not just building a stronger, fitter body but also fostering a healthier, more resilient gut-brain axis. So, the next time you lace up your sneakers for a run or unroll your yoga mat, remember you're doing much more than just burning calories. You're cultivating a garden of health that blooms from the inside out.

TYPES OF EXERCISE FOR GUT HEALTH

When exploring exercise for gut health, we discover a range of benefits beyond toning muscles or shedding pounds. The right types of physical activity can be a powerful ally in nurturing the gut-brain connection, enhancing our overall well-being in the process. Let's explore some of the most effective exercises that can help us achieve a happier gut and a clearer mind.

Aerobic Exercise

First, aerobic exercises, often called cardio, are a fantastic starting point. Think brisk walking, jogging, swimming, or cycling. These activities get the heart pumping and blood flowing, which, in turn, can stimulate food movement through the intestines, reducing constipation and bloating. But the benefits don't stop there. Aerobic exercises have been shown to increase the diversity of gut microbiota, which plays a crucial role in our mental health, immune system, and weight management.

Strength Training

Next, we must recognize the importance of strength training. While it's well-known for building muscle mass and increasing metabolism, lifting weights also contributes to a robust gut. It does so by reducing inflammation and improving the balance of gut bacteria.

Yoga and Pilates

Yoga and Pilates deserve a special mention, too. These aren't just exercises for flexibility and core strength but also fantastic for our digestive system. The various poses and stretches can massage internal organs, helping ease digestion and alleviate gas and bloating. The stress-reducing effects of yoga and Pilates can also lower cortisol levels, which is beneficial since stress is a known factor that can disrupt our gut microbiome.

Walking

Lastly, don't underestimate the power of a good walk. It's simple, but walking is incredibly effective in promoting gut health. It encourages the passing of gas through the digestive system and can help keep things moving smoothly. Plus, it's a great way to clear the mind, reducing stress and anxiety, which, as we've seen, is closely linked to our gut health.

Incorporating a mix of these exercises into our routine can be a game-changer for our gut health and, by extension, our mental well-being. It's not about choosing one over the other but finding a balance that works for you. The key is consistency, listening to your body, and adjusting as needed to support your gut-brain axis in the best way possible.

EXERCISE AND GUT FLORA

Another fascinating aspect of physical activity that deserves our attention is its impact on gut flora. Yes, the trillions of microorganisms in our digestive system are influenced by how much and what type of exercise we do. This connection between exercise regimens and gut flora is not just intriguing; it's a vital piece of the puzzle in understanding the gut-brain axis.

Let's dive a bit deeper. Regular, moderate exercise has been shown to increase the diversity of our gut microbiome. This is a good thing. A more diverse microbiome is often a sign of better gut health, which, in turn, can influence our overall health and even our mood and cognitive functions.

But how exactly does this work? Exercise increases the production of certain substances in our body that help beneficial gut bacteria thrive. For example, physical activity raises the level of butyrate, a short-chain fatty acid that feeds the good bacteria in our gut. This not only helps these beneficial bacteria grow but also reduces inflammation and improves the gut's barrier function, which can prevent harmful substances from leaking into the bloodstream and causing health issues.

Now, you might wonder if all exercises are created equal in the eyes of our gut flora. As we learned earlier, the answer is nuanced. Aerobic exercises like walking, running, and cycling have the most pronounced effect on increasing gut microbiome diversity. However, resistance training is also beneficial, especially for maintaining a healthy body composition, indirectly supporting gut health. The key is consistency and variety. A mix of aerobic and resistance training, performed regularly, is the best recipe for a happy gut.

It's also worth noting that overdoing it can have the opposite effect. Excessive exercise, especially without adequate recovery, can lead to gut dysbiosis, where harmful bacteria outnumber the beneficial ones. This can increase inflammation and negatively affect gut barrier integrity. So, like many things in life, balance is crucial.

Incorporating regular, varied exercise into your routine is not just about building muscle or improving your cardiovascular health; it's also about nurturing your gut flora. By doing so, you're supporting the complex and bidirectional relationship between your gut and your brain, ultimately contributing to both your physical and mental well-being.

CHALLENGES IN STARTING AN EXERCISE ROUTINE

Embarking on a new exercise routine can feel like setting sail into uncharted waters. It's exciting, sure, but it's also fraught with challenges that can make even the most determined of us want to turn the ship around. Let's discuss some of these hurdles to prepare you for the journey ahead. After all, forewarned is forearmed.

First off, there's the issue of time. Finding time for exercise can seem like squeezing water from a stone in a world where our schedules are already bursting at the seams. It's not just about carving out an hour or two for the gym; it's about the commute, the preparation, and the cooldown afterward. The trick here is not to find time but to make it. Consider integrating physical activity into your daily routine in simple ways, like taking the stairs instead of the elevator or going for a walk during your lunch break.

Then, there's the intimidation factor. Gyms can be intimidating places, filled with complicated equipment and people who look like they've been training for marathons since they could walk. Remember, everyone started somewhere, and most people are too focused on their own workouts to pay attention to yours. If the gym's not your scene, there are countless other ways to get active that don't involve a treadmill or weights. Hiking, dancing, swimming, or even gardening can stimulate your heart and benefit your gut-brain axis.

Motivation is another common stumbling block. It's one thing to start an exercise routine and another to stick with it. Motivation tends to wane, especially when results aren't immediate. Setting realistic goals and celebrating small victories can keep you on track. Also, consider finding an exercise buddy. Having someone to share the journey with can make all the difference in keeping you motivated. We'll explore more ways to stay motivated in in the next section.

Lastly, there's the physical aspect. It's normal to experience soreness and fatigue as you begin a new exercise regimen. Listen to your body. Pushing too hard too soon can lead to burnout or injury. Start slow, focus on consistency, and gradually increase the intensity of your workouts. Remember, this is a marathon, not a sprint.

Starting an exercise routine can be challenging. But remember, it's also an opportunity to improve your physical health, mental well-being, and gut health. With some planning, patience, and perseverance, you can overcome these hurdles and find a path to a healthier you.

MAINTAINING MOTIVATION

Embarking on a journey to improve your gut health through exercise is exciting and challenging. The initial burst of enthusiasm can sometimes wane, leaving you searching for the motivation to continue. It's a common scenario, but fear not—maintaining motivation is achievable with the right mindset and strategies.

Firstly, remember why you started. Regular physical activity can enhance this connection, improving your mood, digestion, and immune system. Keep these benefits in mind as a source of inspiration.

Setting realistic goals is crucial. Instead of aiming for immediate, drastic changes, focus on small, achievable milestones. Celebrate each success, no matter how minor it may seem. This approach fosters a sense of accomplishment and propels you forward, step by step.

Variety is the spice of life, and this also applies to exercise routines. Mixing up your activities can prevent boredom and keep things interesting. Whether you try a new fitness class, explore a different hiking trail, or incorporate yoga, variety can reinvigorate your enthusiasm for staying active.

Social support can be a powerful motivator. Joining a community, whether online or in person, connects you with others on similar journeys. Sharing experiences, challenges, and successes can provide encouragement and accountability. Sometimes, knowing you're not alone in your struggles can make all the difference.

Lastly, listen to your body. There will be days when you feel energized and ready to conquer the world and others when rest is what you need most. Respecting your body's signals is vital to a sustainable exercise routine that supports your gut-brain connection without leading to burnout.

Maintaining motivation for exercise in the context of the gut-brain axis is a multifaceted endeavor. It's about setting realistic goals, embracing variety, seeking support, and listening to your body. Remember, this journey is not just about the destination but also about the path you take to get there. No matter how small, each step is a step towards a healthier you.

CASE STUDIES

Let's delve into a couple of success stories that inspire and illuminate the radical impact exercise can have on our gut health.

First, meet Jamie. Jamie's journey began in a place many of us might find familiar: feeling sluggish, mentally foggy, and generally out of sync. The turning point came when Jamie decided to lace up some old running shoes and hit the pavement. Initially, it was a struggle. Breathing was hard, his muscles ached, and the couch never seemed more appealing. But persistence paid off. Over weeks, then months, Jamie noticed something remarkable. The physical changes were expected—more energy, better sleep, a fitter body—but the mental and emotional transformation truly stood out. Alex felt happier, more focused, and surprisingly, less prone to the digestive discomfort that had been a constant annoyance. This wasn't magic; it was science in action. Regular exercise had begun to rebalance Jamie's gut microbiome, leading to improved gut health and, as a result, a happier brain.

Then there's Hannah. Not a running or weightlifting fan, Hannah found joy in dance and yoga. These activities might seem gentle compared to high-intensity workouts. Still, their impact on Hannah's gut-brain axis was anything but mild. Through the rhythmic movements of dance and the mindful stretching of yoga, Hannah experienced a reduction in stress levels, which positively affected her gut health. The bloating and discomfort that used to be daily challenges began to fade, making room for more energy and a newfound sense of inner peace. Hannah's story is a perfect example of how finding the right exercise for you can be a game-changer. It also shows the power of diversity in exercise.

What Jamie and Hannah's stories teach us is meaningful yet simple: the path to improving our gut-brain connection is as unique as we are. It's not about the most intense workout or following the latest fitness trends. It's about finding what moves you, both literally and figuratively. The benefits of exercise extend far beyond the physical, reaching deep into our guts and minds and fostering a sense of well-being that can transform our lives.

As we've journeyed through the science and stories of the gut-brain connection, it's clear that exercise is a powerful ally. Whether you're a runner, a yogi, or someone who finds joy in a brisk walk, the key is to keep moving. Your gut—and your brain—will thank you.

CHAPTER SUMMARY

- Exercise strengthens the gut-brain axis, impacting physical and mental health by promoting a healthy balance of gut microbiota and stimulating the production of beneficial compounds like short-chain fatty acids.

- Physical activity boosts brain health by increasing the production of neurotrophic factors, which support neuron survival and growth, improve cognitive function, and lower the risk of mental health disorders.
- Regular exercise supports a healthier gut environment by reducing the harmful effects of chronic stress, like microbiome disruption and increased gut permeability.
- Aerobic exercises, strength training, yoga, Pilates, and walking are effective activities for nurturing the gut-brain connection. Each offers unique benefits to gut health and overall well-being.
- Consistent, moderate exercise increases gut microbiome diversity, which is linked to better health. In contrast, excessive exercise without proper recovery can negatively impact gut flora balance.
- Challenges in starting an exercise routine include finding time, overcoming gym intimidation, maintaining motivation, and dealing with initial physical discomfort. Still, these can be managed with realistic goal-setting and gradual progression.
- Maintaining motivation for exercise involves remembering the deep-rooted connection between gut health and overall well-being, setting realistic goals, embracing variety in exercise routines, seeking social support, and listening to your body.

CHAPTER 5
SLEEP AND THE GUT-BRAIN CONNECTION

Ah, sleep. It's that golden chain that ties our health and bodies together. Let's dive into why it's particularly crucial when discussing the gut-brain connection.

Imagine your brain and gut as two chatty neighbors over a fence, constantly gossiping back and forth. In this analogy, sleep is like the quality of their phone line. Poor sleep? That's a crackly, barely-there connection. Good sleep? Crystal clear communication.

Research shows that poor sleep can lead to an unhappy gut. This can manifest in several ways, from the more obvious, like bloating and discomfort, to the more subtle, like heightened stress levels and mood changes. It's a two-way street, though. Just as poor sleep can upset our gut, an unhappy gut can make it harder to get a good night's sleep, creating a vicious cycle that's hard to break.

But here's where it gets interesting. When we prioritize sleep, giving ourselves those precious 7-9 hours of quality shut-eye, we're giving our gut-brain communication line a major upgrade. Better sleep leads to a happier, healthier gut, which, in turn, sends positive signals back to the brain, improving our mood, cognitive function, and resilience to stress.

So, how do we ensure this communication line stays open and clear? It starts with the basics: establishing a regular sleep schedule, creating a restful environment free of screens and distractions, and perhaps most importantly, listening to our bodies. They're pretty good at telling us what they need, after all.

In the grand scheme of things, sleep might be one piece of the puzzle, but it's a cornerstone that supports the intricate, fascinating dialogue between our gut and brain. By giving sleep the attention it deserves, we're not just resting our bodies but nurturing our mental and emotional health, one night at a time.

SLEEP DISORDERS AND GUT HEALTH

When we dive into the intricate world of sleep disorders and gut health, we're exploring a realm where the night's rest—or the lack thereof—plays a pivotal role in our digestive well-being. It's a topic that hits home for many, including myself.

It's fascinating to think that the microbes residing in our gut can influence our sleep patterns and vice versa. Research has shown that individuals with sleep disorders often experience changes in their gut microbiome, which can lead to a cascade of health issues beyond just feeling tired.

For instance, poor sleep can disrupt the gut's balance of beneficial and harmful bacteria. This imbalance can contribute to digestive problems, from bloating and discomfort to more severe conditions like irritable bowel syndrome or inflammatory bowel disease. Conversely, a healthy gut can promote better sleep quality by producing and regulating key neurotransmitters and hormones involved in sleep, such as serotonin and melatonin.

Addressing sleep disorders can have a ripple effect, improving our mental and emotional well-being and digestive health. Simple lifestyle changes, like those we'll explore in the next section, can make a big difference. For me, the journey to better sleep was part of my journey to a happier gut. It involved learning to listen to my body's signals, adjusting my diet, and finding stress-reduction techniques that worked for me.

Whether you've struggled with sleep issues, faced digestive discomfort, or are simply interested in optimizing your health, understanding this connection can be a game-changer. It reminds us that our bodies are interconnected systems, and by caring for one part, we're supporting the whole.

THE ROLE OF CIRCADIAN RHYTHMS

Our circadian rhythm plays a pivotal role in the relationship between sleep and the gut-brain connection. Imagine your body as a finely tuned orchestra, with each instrument playing its part in harmony. The circadian rhythms are the conductors, ensuring that every section comes in at the right time and maintaining the balance and flow of the music. This analogy isn't far from the truth when we consider how these rhythms orchestrate the complex interactions between our gut health and brain function, particularly through the regulation of sleep.

Our circadian rhythms are our internal biological clocks. They run on a 24-hour cycle and influence various bodily functions, including hormone release, eating habits, digestion, and sleep-wake cycles. These rhythms are not just a response to the light and darkness we experience but also intertwined with our gut health. The microbes in our gut follow this same circadian pattern. They produce and respond to various signals that affect our brain and, consequently, our sleep.

When our circadian rhythms are in sync, our sleep is more

restorative, and our gut health can flourish, creating a positive feedback loop that benefits our mental and physical health. However, when these rhythms are disrupted, it can lead to a cascade of issues. Poor sleep can alter gut microbiome composition, leading to mood, cognitive function, and overall health changes. Similarly, an unhealthy gut can send signals to the brain that disrupt sleep patterns, creating a vicious cycle that can be hard to break.

We can support the delicate balance between our gut and brain by aligning our lifestyle with our natural biological rhythms—such as maintaining regular sleep schedules, eating consistently, and exposing ourselves to natural light during the day. This, in turn, enhances our sleep quality, mood, and cognitive function, illustrating the influence of our internal biological clock on our overall well-being.

So, as we delve deeper into the connection between sleep and the gut-brain axis, let's not overlook our circadian rhythms. By understanding and respecting these natural cycles, we can harmonize our health, ensuring that each part of our body plays its role perfectly in the symphony of our lives.

PRACTICAL TIPS FOR BETTER SLEEP AND GUT HEALTH

Sleep is a key player in the quest for better gut health. It's a two-way street: just as our gut health can influence our sleep patterns, the quality and quantity of our sleep can have extensive effects on our gut health. Let's explore some practical steps to improve sleep, thereby nurturing a healthier gut-brain connection.

Keep a Consistent Sleep Schedule

Firstly, establishing a consistent sleep schedule is vital. Our bodies thrive on routine. By going to bed and waking up at the same time each day (yes, even on weekends), we can help regulate our internal clock, or circadian rhythm, which in turn can improve our sleep quality. This consistency makes it easier to fall asleep. It promotes a more restful night's sleep, which benefits our gut microbiome.

Pre-Sleep Rituals

Next, consider your pre-sleep rituals. In the hour leading up to bedtime, engage in calming activities to signal to your body that it's time to wind down. This could be reading a book, taking a warm bath, or practicing gentle yoga or meditation. This ritual can help ease the transition between wakefulness and sleep, making it easier to drift off. It's also crucial to limit exposure to screens. This is because the blue light emitted by phones, tablets, and computers can interfere with the production of melatonin, the hormone responsible for sleep.

Set the Right Environment

Your sleeping environment also plays an important role. Ensure your bedroom is conducive to sleep: cool, dark, and quiet. Investing in a comfortable mattress and pillows can also make a significant difference. Consider using blackout curtains, eye masks, earplugs, or listening to white noise if necessary. Your bedroom should be a sleep sanctuary that invites relaxation and restfulness, so keep it free from distractions like TVs and smartphones.

Diet

Dietary habits can also influence sleep quality. Aim to finish eating at least two to three hours before bedtime to give your body time to digest. Be mindful of consuming caffeine and alcohol before bed, as both can disrupt sleep patterns. Instead, consider sipping on herbal tea, such as chamomile, which has been shown to promote relaxation and may improve sleep quality.

Exercise

Regular physical activity is another pillar of good sleep hygiene. Exercise can help you fall asleep faster and enjoy deeper sleep. However, timing is important. Engaging in vigorous exercise too close to bedtime can be stimulating, so aim to complete intense workouts earlier in the day.

Don't Force It

If you're lying in bed, unable to sleep, don't force it. Get up, do something relaxing in low light, and only return to bed when you're feeling sleepy. This helps prevent your bed from being associated with wakefulness.

Seek Help If Needed

Lastly, if sleep issues persist, keeping a sleep diary or consulting with a healthcare professional may be beneficial. Sometimes, underlying conditions such as sleep apnea or anxiety can affect sleep quality and, by extension, gut health. Addressing these issues can lead to improvements in both sleep and overall well-being.

By prioritizing sleep, we're not just giving our bodies the rest they need but also fostering a healthier gut environment. This, in turn, can enhance our mood, cognitive function, and resilience to stress. Remember, improving sleep is a journey, not a sprint. Small, consistent changes can significantly improve sleep quality and gut health, helping you feel better every day. So, here's to better nights ahead!

CASE STUDIES

The following stories illuminate the moving impact of improving sleep quality on gut health and vice versa, providing a deeper understanding of this intricate relationship.

One such story is that of Sarah, a 42-year-old teacher who experienced anxiety alongside her long-standing battle with gastroesophageal reflux disease (GERD). Sarah noticed that her anxiety and stress levels directly influenced her sleep quality and GERD symptoms. With the help of cognitive-behavioral therapy and dietary adjustments, Sarah learned to manage her stress and anxiety more effectively. As her mental well-being improved, she found that her sleep became more restorative, and her GERD symptoms lessened noticeably. Sarah's experience shows the multifaceted nature of the gut-brain connection and the role of mental health in this dynamic.

Then, we have the story of Ben, a 28-year-old athlete who suffered from sleep apnea and noticed its impact on his digestive health. Ben's disrupted sleep patterns due to sleep apnea affected his energy levels and overall well-being. After undergoing a sleep study and receiving appropriate treatment for sleep apnea, Ben experienced a notable improvement in his sleep quality. This improvement had a ripple effect, enhancing his digestive health and overall performance. Ben's case highlights the importance of addressing sleep disorders in the context of gut health and the gut-brain connection.

These stories exemplify the intricate relationship between sleep and gut health, showing how improvements in one area can lead to positive outcomes in the other. They are a testament to the power of holistic approaches in addressing the complexities of the gut-brain connection, offering hope and guidance for those navigating similar challenges.

CHAPTER SUMMARY

- Sleep is crucial for maintaining a healthy gut-brain connection, acting as the communication line between the two.
- Poor sleep can disrupt gut health, leading to issues like bloating, stress, and mood changes, creating a vicious cycle.
- Prioritizing 7-9 hours of quality sleep can improve gut health, mood, cognitive function, and stress resilience.
- Sleep disorders and gut health are interconnected, with sleep issues often leading to changes in the gut microbiome and vice versa.
- Circadian rhythms play a key role in regulating sleep and gut health, with disruptions affecting both negatively.
- Practical steps for better sleep include establishing a consistent sleep schedule, creating a restful environment, and managing diet and exercise.

CHAPTER 6
HOLISTIC APPROACHES TO GUT HEALTH

Let me share a bit of my own story. A few years back, I found myself caught in the relentless grip of digestive issues, which, as I later learned, were intricately linked to my mental well-being. The conventional route provided relief, yes, but it was often fleeting. It wasn't until I embraced a more integrative approach, combining the wisdom of traditional medicine with the insights of alternative practices, that I began to see a lasting change.

This section delves into how blending traditional medical practices with alternative medicine can create a comprehensive approach to gut health.

Traditional medicine, with its deep roots in scientific research and evidence-based treatments, offers a solid foundation for addressing the physical aspects of gut health. It's where we turn for diagnostics, medication, and interventions that have been tested and proven over time. Yet, it often focuses on treating symptoms rather than the underlying causes.

On the other hand, alternative medicine encompasses a broad spectrum of practices, including herbal remedies, acupuncture, yoga, and meditation, to name a few. While sometimes lacking in rigorous scientific validation compared to traditional medicine, these approaches offer invaluable insights into the holistic management of health. They emphasize the interconnectedness of the mind, body, and spirit, advocating for preventative measures and natural healing.

By combining the strengths of both worlds, we can create a more nuanced and effective strategy for managing gut health. For example, while traditional medicine can alleviate symptoms through medication, alternative practices can offer stress reduction techniques that address the root causes of gut issues. Similarly, dietary recommendations can be enhanced with herbal supplements known to support gut health, providing a more comprehensive approach to healing.

Integrating traditional and alternative medicine doesn't mean choosing one over the other; it means understanding and applying the best of both to achieve optimal health.

As we explore this holistic approach, remember that the journey to gut health is as much about healing as it is about discovery. It's a process of learning to listen to your body, understanding its signals, and responding with a blend of science and nature. My journey taught me that healing is not just about the absence of illness but about achieving balance and well-being that encompasses the whole person.

HERBAL REMEDIES AND SUPPLEMENTS

Herbal remedies have been the backbone of traditional medicine for centuries, offering a natural path to healing. When it comes to the gut-brain connection, certain herbs stand out for their potential to soothe the gut, thereby influencing our mental well-being. Take, for instance, ginger. This root, known for its zesty kick, is not just a culinary delight but also a potent anti-inflammatory agent. It can help ease digestive discomfort, which, in turn, may alleviate stress and anxiety.

Another star in the herbal galaxy is peppermint. Beyond its refreshing scent, peppermint oil has been shown to relax the muscles of the digestive tract, easing symptoms of irritable bowel syndrome — a condition that can impact one's quality of life and mental health.

But it's not just herbs that hold the key to gut health. Supplements, particularly probiotics, have taken center stage in recent years. These beneficial bacteria are crucial for maintaining a healthy gut microbiome. By supporting our gut flora, probiotics can be a valuable tool in enhancing our gut-brain connection.

Finding the right herbal remedy or supplement is a personal journey influenced by individual health needs and conditions. For some, a daily probiotic supplement can make a world of difference. Others may find relief in a cup of chamomile tea before bed.

It's also important to remember that natural doesn't always mean safe. Interactions between herbal remedies and conventional medications can occur, and not all supplements are created equal. Quality and purity can vary widely, making it essential to choose products from reputable sources and consult with a healthcare professional before starting any new supplement regimen.

Integrating herbal remedies and supplements into our approach to gut health offers a bridge between traditional wisdom and modern science. It's a testament to the power of nature in supporting our well-being, reminding us that sometimes, the simplest solutions can be found in the world around us.

ACUPUNCTURE

Acupuncture is a fascinating and ancient practice that has garnered attention for its potential benefits on the gut-brain axis. Originating from traditional Chinese medicine, acupuncture involves the insertion of thin needles into specific points on the body. It's believed to stimulate the body's energy flow, or Qi, and bring about healing and balance. But how does this relate to our gut health and, by extension, our mental well-being?

Research suggests that acupuncture can help regulate the digestive system, alleviate stress, and reduce inflammation – all of which are beneficial for gut health. By targeting specific acupuncture points, practitioners aim to restore balance and promote the body's natural healing processes. For instance, specific points on the body are believed to enhance gastrointestinal muscle contraction and relaxation and reduce gastric acid secretion, which can help alleviate symptoms of conditions like irritable bowel syndrome and acid reflux.

Acupuncture's ability to modulate the stress response is particularly relevant to gut health. Through its calming effect on the nervous system, acupuncture can help mitigate the impact of stress on the gut, thereby improving overall digestive function and comfort.

Acupuncture's holistic approach, which considers physical and emotional health, aligns perfectly with this concept. By addressing gut health, acupuncture can also improve mood and cognitive function. It offers a compelling and integrative solution for those seeking to enhance the health of their gut and brain.

While the scientific community continues to explore the mechanisms behind acupuncture's effects on gut health, anecdotal evidence and a growing body of research support its potential as a valuable component of an integrative approach to digestive and mental well-being. As with any alternative therapy, it's important to consult with healthcare professionals and consider acupuncture as part of a comprehensive health plan tailored to individual needs and conditions.

MASSAGE THERAPY

While massage therapy is widely recognized for its ability to relax and rejuvenate the mind and body, its benefits extend deep into the gut, influencing our digestive well-being in many ways.

Massage therapy can indirectly support gut health by reducing stress and promoting relaxation. The physical manipulation of body tissues helps to relieve tension in the abdominal area, improving circulation and encouraging the movement of digestive contents. This can be particularly beneficial for those suffering from conditions like constipation or irritable bowel syndrome, where stress and muscle tension play an integral role.

Moreover, massage therapy stimulates the parasympathetic nervous system—the part of our nervous system that governs the 'rest and digest' response. Activation of this system encourages the body to focus on digestion and nutrient absorption, which is essential for maintaining a healthy gut microbiome.

But how do you incorporate massage therapy into a gut health regimen? It's simpler than you might think. Seeking a professional massage therapist who understands the intricacies of the gut-brain connection can be a good start. They can tailor massage techniques to target the abdominal area, promoting relaxation and supporting digestive function. Self-massage techniques can also be learned and practiced at home, offering a convenient and cost-effective way to reap the benefits.

Massage therapy offers a unique and integrative path to supporting gut health. It leverages the power of touch to heal and harmonize the gut-brain connection. However, it's important to note that massage therapy is not a standalone cure for digestive ailments. It works best when integrated into a holistic approach to health that includes a balanced diet, regular exercise, and stress management techniques. Always consult a healthcare provider before starting any new treatment, especially if you have existing health conditions.

YOGA

Yoga offers a gentle yet powerful approach to fostering a harmonious gut-brain connection. This ancient practice, rooted in the integration of mind, body, and spirit, has been shown to positively affect gut health and overall well-being.

Yoga, with its myriad poses (asanas), breathing techniques (pranayama), and meditation practices, serves not just as a physical exercise but as a holistic practice that addresses stress, one of the primary culprits behind gut imbalances. Stress, as we've explored, can wreak havoc on our digestive system, leading to a cascade of issues that affect our mental and physical health. Yoga's ability to mitigate stress is a key factor in its beneficial effects on gut health.

Practicing yoga encourages the activation of the parasympathetic nervous system. This activation is crucial for maintaining a healthy gut, as it enhances digestive function and fosters a state of calm within the body. Through specific poses that massage and stimulate the abdominal organs, yoga can improve digestion and facilitate the elimination of toxins, further contributing to gut health.

Moreover, yoga's emphasis on mindfulness and present-moment awareness can lead to more mindful eating habits. This heightened awareness can help individuals tune into their body's hunger and fullness signals, promoting a healthier relationship with food and preventing gastrointestinal distress caused by overeating or eating too quickly.

Yoga is accessible to everyone, regardless of age or fitness level, making it an inclusive option for improving gut health. Whether it's a gentle restorative class, a more dynamic vinyasa flow, or a focused pranayama practice, each style of yoga offers unique benefits for the gut-brain axis. It's about finding the practice that resonates with you and your body's needs.

Yoga offers a path to improved gut health by fostering balance and harmony within, illustrating the interconnectedness of our mind, body, and spirit.

Incorporating yoga into your routine can be as simple as starting with a few minutes each day, gradually building up as you become more comfortable and attuned to its effects on your body. The beauty of yoga lies in its adaptability; it can be practiced anywhere, from the comfort of your home to a local park or a dedicated yoga studio.

CHAPTER SUMMARY

- Integrative approaches to gut health combine traditional and alternative medicine, offering a holistic wellness pathway that addresses physical symptoms and underlying causes.
- Traditional medicine provides a solid foundation for addressing gut health through diagnostics and evidence-based treatments. However, it often focuses on symptoms rather than causes.
- Alternative medicine, including herbal remedies, acupuncture, yoga, and meditation, offers insights

into holistic health management. It emphasizes the interconnectedness of mind, body, and spirit.
- Combining traditional and alternative approaches allows for a nuanced strategy to address root causes of gut issues, such as stress, through complementary practices like stress reduction techniques and dietary supplements.
- Herbal remedies and supplements, like ginger and probiotics, are powerful in supporting gut health, but quality and interactions with medications should be considered.
- Acupuncture and massage therapy have potential benefits on the gut-brain axis. They can regulate digestion, reduce stress, and improve mental well-being as part of an integrative health plan.
- Yoga offers a gentle yet powerful approach to boosting the gut-brain connection through its power to reduce stress, activate the parasympathetic nervous system, and practice mindfulness.

CHAPTER 7
MENTAL HEALTH AND THE GUT

It's fascinating how the intricate dialogue between our gut and brain can impact our mental health. Let's dive into this relationship and understand how it impacts those dealing with mental health conditions like depression and anxiety.

For individuals experiencing depression or anxiety, this gut-brain dialogue can sometimes be out of balance. Research suggests that an imbalance in the gut microbiota may contribute to the development or exacerbation of these mental health conditions. As we explored in previous chapters, certain strains of bacteria can produce neurotransmitters like serotonin and gamma-aminobutyric acid, which are critical for regulating mood. A deficiency in these neurotransmitters is often linked to depression and anxiety.

Moreover, the gut microbiome can influence the body's stress response system, known as the hypothalamic-pituitary-adrenal (HPA) axis. An imbalance in the gut microbiota can lead to an overactive HPA axis, resulting in higher levels of stress and anxiety. This is why stress management techniques, such as mindfulness and meditation, help calm the mind and positively affect gut health, creating a beneficial feedback loop.

Emerging treatments focusing on the gut-brain axis offer new hope for those struggling with depression and anxiety. Probiotics, prebiotics, and dietary changes are being explored as potential interventions to restore balance in the gut microbiota and, by extension, improve mental health outcomes.

The connection between the gut and brain offers exciting avenues for understanding and treating depression and anxiety. By nurturing our gut microbiome through diet, stress management, and possibly probiotics, we can transform our mental health. This burgeoning field of research holds promise for developing more holistic approaches to mental health care, emphasizing the importance of the gut-brain connection in achieving emotional well-being.

THE ROLE OF INFLAMMATION

In the intricate dance between our mental health and gut, inflammation plays a leading role, often dictating the rhythm and pace at which our bodies and minds interact. It's a concept that might seem complex at first glance, but let's break it down into simpler terms to understand how inflammation impacts our overall well-being.

Think about all of the trillions of bacteria living in your gut. The gut has its own ecosystem that must be balanced for everything to run smoothly. However, when unwanted invaders, such as harmful bacteria or viruses, enter this ecosystem, they can disrupt the peace. This disruption triggers an immune response, leading to inflammation. While inflammation is the body's way of protecting itself, chronic inflammation can become problematic, acting like a city under constant siege.

This is where the gut-brain connection comes into play.

When the gut is inflamed, it sends signals to the brain, which can lead to changes in mood, behavior, and cognitive functions.

Inflammation in the gut has been linked to several mental health conditions, including depression and anxiety. Studies have shown that people with these conditions often have higher levels of specific inflammatory markers. This doesn't mean inflammation causes these conditions outright, but it suggests a powerful relationship between them.

So, how do you manage inflammation to support mental health? The answer lies in a combination of diet, lifestyle changes, and, in some cases, medication. Foods rich in anti-inflammatory properties, such as omega-3 fatty acids found in fish and antioxidants in fruits and vegetables, can help reduce inflammation. Regular exercise, adequate sleep, and stress management techniques like mindfulness and meditation also play a crucial role in keeping inflammation at bay.

Understanding the role of inflammation in the gut-brain connection enables us to find new ways to treat and manage mental health conditions. It emphasizes the importance of a holistic approach to health, where caring for our gut is essential for mental well-being.

PREVENTATIVE MEASURES

In the realm of mental health, the adage *"prevention is better than cure"* holds a transformative truth. Taking proactive steps to maintain gut health is not just about physical well-being but is intrinsically linked to our mental state. The gut-brain connection offers a unique lens through which we can understand and mitigate the risks of mental health issues before they take root.

First and foremost, diet plays a pivotal role in this preventive approach. As we explored earlier, a balanced diet rich in fiber, vegetables, fruits, and fermented foods supports a diverse and robust microbiome, which, in turn, positively influences our mental health. It's not just about what we eat but how our body interacts with these foods, breaking them down and allowing the beneficial bacteria in our gut to thrive. These bacteria produce short-chain fatty acids and neurotransmitters that can impact our mood and cognitive functions, illustrating the direct line of communication between our gut and brain. On the flip side, a diet high in processed foods and sugars can lead to an imbalance in gut bacteria, potentially exacerbating mental health issues like depression and anxiety.

Probiotics and prebiotics play a starring role in this narrative. Probiotics, the beneficial bacteria found in fermented foods like yogurt, kefir, and sauerkraut, can help restore balance to the gut microbiome. Prebiotics, on the other hand, are the dietary fibers that feed these beneficial bacteria. Integrating these into your diet can support gut health and, by extension, mental health.

Regular physical activity is another cornerstone of preventive measures. Exercise promotes the growth of beneficial and diverse gut bacteria. This, in turn, can enhance the production of mood-regulating neurotransmitters, providing a natural boost to our mental well-being. Whether it's a brisk walk, a yoga session, or a more intense workout, the key is consistency and finding joy in the movement.

Stress management is equally crucial. Chronic stress can wreak havoc on our gut, disrupting the delicate balance of our microbiome and leading to inflammation, which is often linked to various mental health conditions. Techniques such as mindfulness, meditation, and yoga not only help manage stress but also have been shown to positively impact gut health. These practices can reduce inflammation and improve the diversity of the gut microbiome, creating a more favorable environment for mental health.

As we explored in earlier chapters, quality sleep is essential for maintaining a healthy microbiome and gut-brain axis. Disruptions in our sleep patterns can affect our microbiome and increase our susceptibility to stress and inflammation, creating a vicious cycle that impacts our mental health. Establishing a regular sleep routine and creating a conducive sleep environment are simple yet effective strategies to enhance gut health and mental well-being.

Lastly, fostering social connections and engaging in activities that bring joy and fulfillment can improve our gut health and mental state. Happiness, laughter, and positive social interactions can influence our gut bacteria, demonstrating the interconnectedness of our emotional state, gut health, and overall well-being.

In conclusion, the journey to mental health through the gateway of gut health is paved with a holistic approach encompassing diet, exercise, stress management, sleep, and social well-being. By adopting these preventative measures, we nurture our gut microbiome and fortify our mental resilience, opening up a path to a happier, healthier life.

CASE STUDIES

In the realm of mental health and the gut, the stories of transformation are as compelling as they are inspiring. Among these tales, one in particular stands out—not because it's mine, but because it mirrors the experiences of many.

A few years ago, I found myself in a relentless battle with anxiety. It was a constant, unwelcome companion that made every day a challenge. Conventional treatments provided some relief, but when I stumbled upon the concept of the gut-brain connection, I found a turning point. Skeptical yet desperate, I decided to try it, overhauling my diet and focusing on gut health. The change was gradual but undeniable. As my gut health improved, so did my mental state. It was a personal victory that fueled my passion for this very topic.

But my story is just one of many. Take, for example, my friend Mia, a 35-year-old teacher who suffered from debilitating depression for over a decade. After countless medications and therapy sessions, she turned to her diet as a last resort. Within months of adopting a gut-friendly diet rich in probiotics, prebiotics, and nutrient-dense foods, Mia began to experience a lightness she hadn't felt in years. Her depression didn't vanish overnight, but it became manageable, allowing her to reclaim her life.

Then there's Michael, a veteran with PTSD, who found solace not in medication but in meditation and a gut-centric lifestyle. Combining mindfulness practices and a diet focused on healing his gut helped alleviate his symptoms to a degree he never thought possible. Michael's journey shows the power of integrative approaches in healing the mind and body.

These stories, including my own, are not anomalies. They are evidence of a paradigm shift in our understanding of mental health. Once a fringe theory, the gut-brain connection is now at the forefront of holistic health approaches. It's a reminder that the answers we seek for our most complex problems sometimes lie within us—specifically, our gut.

These stories remind us that transformation is within reach with the proper knowledge and tools. Whether through diet, exercise, mindfulness, or a combination of approaches, the journey to better mental health begins in the gut. And as my own experience has shown, it's a journey well worth taking.

CHAPTER SUMMARY

- The gut-brain connection is increasingly recognized as crucial in understanding and treating depression and anxiety, with the microbiome playing a significant role in this relationship.
- Imbalances in gut microbiota can contribute to the development or exacerbation of depression and anxiety, with certain bacteria affecting neurotransmitter levels like serotonin and GABA.
- The gut microbiome influences the body's stress response system, affecting stress and anxiety levels and highlighting the importance of stress management techniques.
- Inflammation in the gut, often resulting from an imbalance in microbiota, is linked to mental health conditions like depression and anxiety, suggesting a holistic approach to treatment.
- Diet is pivotal in maintaining a healthy gut-brain connection, with fiber-rich foods promoting a healthy microbiome and processed foods contributing to dysbiosis and mental health issues.
- Emerging treatments focusing on the gut-brain axis, such as probiotics, prebiotics, and dietary changes, show promise in improving mental health outcomes.
- Practical gut health interventions, including diet modifications, stress management, exercise, and sleep, can enhance mental health by supporting a healthy gut microbiome.

CHAPTER 8
CHILDREN AND THE GUT-BRAIN CONNECTION

It's easy to imagine the gut-brain connection as a complex conversation happening in adults. But let's shift our focus to where this intricate dialogue begins: in the early years of a child's life. The foundation of a child's gut health and its impact on brain development is a fascinating journey that starts much earlier than many realize.

From the moment a baby is born, they are introduced to a world of bacteria. Yes, bacteria - but not all of it is bad. In fact, this initial exposure plays a crucial role in shaping the baby's gut microbiome, which influences their brain development and overall health. It's a delicate balance that begins with the method of birth. Babies born through vaginal delivery are coated in a layer of beneficial bacteria as they pass through the birth canal. This natural process kick-starts the baby's immune system and gut flora development. On the other hand, babies born via cesarean section miss out on this initial bacterial bath, which can lead to differences in their gut microbiome.

Breastfeeding further contributes to the development of a healthy gut. Breast milk is not just food; it's a complex cocktail of nutrients, antibodies, and prebiotics that nourish the baby and promote the growth of beneficial gut bacteria. This, in turn, supports the baby's immune system and brain development. It's fascinating to think that something as simple as feeding can have such a powerful impact on a child's health and development.

Let me share a little story that brings this all closer to home. When my nephew was born, he faced some challenges that required him to be delivered via a cesarean section. Having read about the importance of early gut health, my sister was determined to breastfeed. It wasn't easy, but she persisted, encouraged by the thought that she was helping to lay the foundation for his future health and well-being. Watching her dedication and understanding the science behind it made me appreciate the incredible impact of these early interactions on a child's life even more.

As children grow, their diet plays a more important role in shaping their gut microbiome. Solid foods introduce new bacteria, further diversifying their gut flora. This diversity is key to a healthy gut, supporting brain health and cognitive development. It's a reminder of the importance of a balanced, nutritious diet from the earliest stages of life.

Understanding the gut-brain connection in children isn't just about appreciating the complexity of human biology. It's about recognizing the influence of early life experiences and choices on a child's health and development. From the method of birth to the first foods they eat, these early decisions lay the foundation for a child's future, influencing everything from their immune system to their mental health.

The journey of the gut-brain connection begins not in adulthood but in the earliest days of childhood. As we continue exploring this connection, let's not forget the importance of nurturing our children's gut health from the very start.

DIETARY IMPACTS ON CHILDREN

When we discuss the diets of children, especially in the context of the gut-brain connection, we're entering a world where every bite matters. It's not just about avoiding a sugar rush or ensuring they eat their greens. It's about understanding how the foods children consume can influence their mood, behavior, and cognitive development. Let's unpack this, shall we?

Consider the standard diet of many children today: high in processed foods, sugars, and artificial additives. These can disrupt the delicate balance of the gut microbiome, leading to inflammation and altering the production of those crucial neurotransmitters. It's not just about an upset stomach; it's about an upset system that can lead to mood swings, increased anxiety, and difficulties with focus and learning.

Conversely, a diet rich in whole foods, fibers, and fermented foods can support a healthy microbiome. Foods like fruits, vegetables, whole grains, and lean proteins provide the nutrients that beneficial gut bacteria thrive on. Fermented foods introduce helpful probiotics into the gut, helping to maintain that critical balance. It's like laying down a solid foundation for a house; you can create a stable and supportive structure with the right building blocks.

But it's not just about the physical health benefits. A balanced diet can also improve children's emotional regulation and cognitive function. Studies have shown that children with healthier diets tend to have better focus, memory, and problem-solving skills. They're also more likely to have a positive outlook on life, showing less aggression and distress. By nourishing the gut, we also nourish the mind.

So, what's the takeaway for parents and caregivers? It's simple yet powerful: the food choices we make for our children can significantly shape their mental and physical health. By choosing whole, nutrient-rich foods and minimizing processed items, we're not just feeding their bodies but their brains. And in doing so, we're giving them the best possible start in life, setting them up for a future where they can thrive mentally and physically. Making the right dietary choices for our children could be the key to unlocking their full potential.

BEHAVIORAL ISSUES AND THE GUT

Imagine a child; let's call her Lily. Lily's diet is heavy on processed foods and sugars and lacks the diversity of nutrients her growing body and brain need. Over time, Lily starts to show signs of hyperactivity and struggles with concentration at school. Her parents are puzzled and concerned, seeking answers and solutions to help their daughter.

Here's where the gut-brain connection comes into play. Our gut is often called our "second brain" for good reason. It's home to a vast network of neurons and a complex microbiome communicating directly with our brain.

In Lily's case, her diet is impacting the balance of her gut microbiome, affecting the production and regulation of neurotransmitters and leading to behavioral issues. It's a chain reaction that starts with what's on her plate.

Research has shown that children with a healthier, more diverse diet tend to have a more balanced gut microbiome, supporting physical, emotional, and behavioral well-being.

But it's not just about adding or removing certain foods. It's about understanding the unique needs of each child's body and how it reacts to different foods. Some children might be more sensitive to food additives and sugar than others. This sensitivity can manifest in various ways, including behavioral changes.

So, what happened to Lily? With guidance, her parents

began to introduce more whole foods into her diet, cutting down on processed foods and sugars. They also included probiotic-rich foods to help support her gut health. Over time, they noticed a big improvement in her behavior and concentration levels.

Lily's story is just one example of how the gut-brain connection can influence children's behavior. It highlights the importance of considering diet as part of the approach to managing behavioral issues.

The gut-brain connection in children is a fascinating and complex relationship that can profoundly impact their behavior. By nurturing the gut with a healthy, balanced diet, we can support not just their physical growth but also their emotional and behavioral development.

PARENTAL GUIDANCE AND SUPPORT

Navigating the complex world of the gut-brain connection in children can feel daunting. Yet, understanding this intricate relationship leads to a realm of interventions and strategies that can enhance a child's well-being. Parents and caregivers hold a unique position of influence that can significantly impact a child's gut health and, by extension, their mental and emotional well-being. This section offers guidance and support as you embark on this journey with your child.

First and foremost, understanding the basics of the gut-brain axis is crucial. It's like knowing the rules of the game before you start playing. This connection means what happens in the gut can affect the brain and vice versa. It's simple, but the implications are profound. This book provides the foundational knowledge you need to navigate this field.

Now, let's talk about practical steps. Begin by observing your child's diet. Are they getting enough fiber, fruits, and vegetables? These foods are not just "good for the gut" but the secret ingredients for a happier, more balanced mood. Consider making mealtime an adventure, exploring new foods together, and making it a fun, educational experience rather than a battleground. A diet rich in whole foods, fruits, vegetables, and fiber can foster a healthy microbiome in children. This, in turn, supports cognitive functions and emotional well-being.

Physical activity is another cornerstone of supporting the gut-brain axis in children. Regular exercise improves gut motility and health and boosts mood and cognitive functions by releasing endorphins and other neurotransmitters. This doesn't mean signing up for every sports team available; instead, find activities your child enjoys. It could be as simple as a family walk or bike ride. The goal is to get moving and have fun doing it.

We know that quality sleep is essential for both gut health and brain function. Establishing a consistent bedtime routine, ensuring the sleeping environment is conducive to rest, and limiting screen time before bed can help improve sleep quality. This, in turn, supports the gut-brain connection by allowing your child to get the restorative sleep their body needs to repair and regenerate overnight.

Stress management is equally important. Much like adults, children can experience stress, which can negatively impact their gut health and, by extension, their brain function. Encourage activities that promote relaxation and mindfulness, such as yoga or meditation, suitable for their age. Even simple breathing exercises can make a big difference. It's about creating a calm environment where your child feels safe and supported.

Lastly, fostering a supportive and understanding environment is vital. Children thrive in environments where they feel safe, loved, and understood. This emotional support can positively influence their gut health and mental well-being. Open communication, active listening, and empathy can go a long way in supporting a child's gut-brain connection.

Remember, you're not alone in this. Seeking advice from healthcare professionals who understand the gut-brain link can provide you with tailored strategies that suit your child's needs. And most importantly, your involvement and support can make all the difference. By being proactive and informed, you can help pave the way for a healthier gut and a happier, more resilient child better equipped to navigate life's challenges. Remember, small changes can make a big difference in a child's life.

CASE STUDIES

Let's delve into a couple of case studies highlighting the transformative power of understanding and nurturing the gut-brain connection in young lives.

First, we meet Emma, a seven-year-old girl who struggles with severe anxiety and digestive issues. Emma's parents were perplexed by her frequent stomach aches and reluctance to attend school. After numerous visits to pediatricians and specialists, the link between Emma's anxiety and her gut health began to emerge. A holistic approach was adopted, focusing on a diet rich in whole foods, probiotics, and prebiotics to support her gut flora. Additionally, Emma began therapy to address her anxiety, including techniques for stress management. Remarkably, as Emma's gut health improved, so did her anxiety levels. This story underscores the bidirectional relationship between the gut and the brain, highlighting how addressing one can beneficially impact the other.

Next, consider the story of Theo, a ten-year-old boy with attention deficit hyperactivity disorder (ADHD). Traditional medication provided some relief but came with undesirable side effects. Theo's parents sought alternative strategies and learned about the potential role of gut health in managing ADHD symptoms. They revamped Theo's diet, eliminating processed foods and sugars while incorporating omega-3 fatty acids, fiber, and fermented foods. Over several months, Theo's focus and behavior improved noticeably. His parents and teachers noted a remarkable change in his ability to concentrate and overall mood. This case illustrates the potential of dietary interventions in managing neurological and behavioral conditions, offering hope for less reliance on medication.

These stories are more than anecdotes; they are beacons of hope for families navigating similar challenges. They reveal the importance of considering the gut-brain connection in children's health and the potential of integrative approaches to foster well-being. As research in this field continues to evolve, it's clear that nurturing the gut-brain axis from a young age can have deep-rooted implications for mental and physical health. These stories not only provide insight into the transformative power of the gut-brain connection but also offer practical strategies that can make a big difference in children's lives.

CHAPTER SUMMARY

- The gut-brain connection begins in early childhood, significantly impacting a child's brain development and overall health.
- Babies born through vaginal delivery receive beneficial bacteria, while those born via cesarean section may have different gut microbiomes.
- Breastfeeding plays a crucial role in developing a healthy gut by providing nutrients, antibodies, and prebiotics.

- The introduction of solid foods diversifies a child's gut flora, emphasizing the importance of a balanced, nutritious diet from early on.
- Dietary choices, including whole foods and minimizing processed items, shape a child's mental and physical health.
- The gut microbiome affects children's mood, behavior, and cognitive development, with diet playing a pivotal role in maintaining a healthy gut-brain connection.
- Strategies to support the gut-brain connection in children include a healthy diet, physical activity, quality sleep, stress management, and emotional support.

CHAPTER 9
AGING AND THE GUT-BRAIN AXIS

Our bodies undergo many changes as we age, and our gut health is no exception. The connection between our gut and our brain evolves with age.

One of the biggest changes we experience as we get older is a change in the composition of our gut microbiota. This community of bacteria, viruses, fungi, and other microorganisms in our digestive system shifts in diversity and abundance. These changes can have far-reaching effects on our health. They can potentially contribute to age-related conditions such as decreased cognitive function, mood disorders, and a weakened immune system.

Why does this happen? Our gut microbiota changes due to several factors. Dietary habits, lifestyle choices, exposure to medications (especially antibiotics), and the natural decline in our digestive system's functionality all play a part. The reduced production of stomach acid and digestive enzymes, for example, can affect the breakdown and absorption of nutrients, which in turn impacts the composition of our microbiota.

Moreover, the integrity of the gut barrier often diminishes with age, a condition we discovered earlier called leaky gut. This can lead to increased intestinal permeability, allowing substances that should be contained within the gut to escape into the bloodstream. This escape can trigger inflammation and immune responses, potentially exacerbating chronic conditions and impacting brain health through inflammatory pathways.

COGNITIVE DECLINE AND THE MICROBIOME

Recent research has begun to shed light on how the microbiome can influence the aging brain, potentially affecting our susceptibility to cognitive decline.

The gut microbiome is incredibly dynamic. As we grow older, the diversity of our gut bacteria tends to decrease, which can have far-reaching effects on our health. This reduction in microbial diversity is associated with several age-related conditions, including cognitive decline and neurodegenerative diseases like Alzheimer's and Parkinson's.

But how exactly does the microbiome influence our brain health as we age? It's all about communication. The gut-brain axis allows for constant dialogue between our gut microbes and brain, primarily through the vagus nerve, immune system, and various metabolic pathways. This communication is crucial for maintaining brain health. A decrease in these beneficial microbes can lead to increased inflammation, a known risk factor for cognitive decline.

Moreover, an imbalance in the neurotransmitters produced by the gut microbiome, such as serotonin and dopamine, can contribute to the development of psychiatric and neurodegenerative disorders.

So, what can we do to support our microbiome and, by extension, our cognitive health as we age? The answer lies in lifestyle choices that promote a healthy, diverse gut microbiome. As we explored in earlier chapters, a diet rich in fiber, fruits, vegetables, and fermented foods can encourage the growth of beneficial gut bacteria. Regular physical activity, adequate sleep, and stress management techniques like mindfulness and meditation can also positively impact our microbiome and overall brain health.

The connection between the microbiome and cognitive decline is a complex but crucial area of study in understanding the aging process. By nurturing our gut health through mindful lifestyle choices, we can support our cognitive function and quality of life as we age.

NUTRITIONAL NEEDS AS WE AGE

Our nutritional needs evolve as our body ages. Maintaining a diet that supports gut health becomes increasingly crucial, given its impact on the brain and overall well-being. Let's recap some of the nutritional strategies we explored earlier and how they can be adapted as we get older.

The digestive system becomes less efficient with age. This reduced efficiency can lead to issues like poor nutrient absorption, which in turn can affect cognitive function and mental health. Therefore, a diet rich in fiber is paramount. Fiber aids digestion and helps maintain a healthy gut microbiome, which is vital for cognitive health and preventing inflammation that can lead to chronic diseases.

Hydration is another crucial aspect of nutrition. The body's sense of thirst diminishes with age, making dehydration a common issue among older adults. Dehydration can exacerbate cognitive problems and negatively affect gut health. Thus, ensuring adequate fluid intake is as crucial as a balanced diet.

Omega-3 fatty acids, found in fish, flaxseeds, and walnuts,

are also essential when we age. These fats are known for their anti-inflammatory properties and role in maintaining brain health. They can help protect against cognitive decline and support the overall health of the gut-brain axis.

Antioxidant-rich foods, such as fruits and vegetables, are critical in combating oxidative stress, which increases with age. These foods can help protect the brain and the digestive system from damage caused by free radicals.

Probiotics and prebiotics should not be overlooked. These can be found in fermented foods like yogurt, kefir, and sauerkraut or dietary supplements. They help maintain a healthy balance of gut bacteria, which is crucial for digestion, nutrient absorption, and immune function. A healthy gut microbiome is linked to reduced risks of mood disorders, which can be particularly beneficial for older people who may be prone to feelings of loneliness and depression.

Lastly, it's essential to consider the practical aspects of nutrition as we get older. Issues such as dental health problems, decreased appetite, and side effects from medication can make eating and absorbing nutrients more challenging. Tailoring our diet to accommodate these changes—such as opting for softer, nutrient-dense foods and ensuring meals are appealing and easy to prepare—can improve health and well-being.

We should consider what choices we can make to support the gut-brain axis as we reach the later years of life. A diet that emphasizes hydration, fiber, omega-3 fatty acids, antioxidants, and probiotics can help mitigate the effects of aging on the body and the brain. By addressing these nutritional needs, we can support not only our physical health but our mental and emotional well-being, too.

LIFESTYLE ADJUSTMENTS

We now know that the connection between our gut and brain becomes even more crucial as we enter the later stages of life. Recognizing this, it becomes essential to consider lifestyle adjustments that can support and nurture this vital connection. Understanding how to nurture this connection can be a game-changer in aging gracefully. Let's explore some preventative strategies that can help maintain a healthy gut-brain axis as we age.

First and foremost, diet plays a pivotal role. As we explored in the last section, a balanced diet rich in fiber, vegetables, fruits, and lean proteins can support gut health and, by extension, brain health. Incorporating fermented foods like yogurt, kefir, and sauerkraut can also introduce beneficial probiotics into the digestive system, fostering a healthy microbiome. It's equally important to stay hydrated. Water aids digestion and helps maintain the balance of good bacteria in the gut.

Physical activity is another cornerstone of supporting the gut-brain axis during aging. We've established that regular exercise benefits the heart and muscles and promotes a healthy gut. Even gentle activities like walking or tai chi can stimulate the movement of food through the digestive system and reduce inflammation, both of which are beneficial for gut health.

Lastly, social connections and mental stimulation play a role in maintaining a healthy gut-brain axis. Engaging in social activities, learning new skills, and pursuing hobbies can reduce stress and challenge your brain, which can, in turn, positively affect gut health. It's about keeping both your mind and your gut engaged and active.

Incorporating these lifestyle adjustments can initially seem daunting, but even small changes can make a difference. Start small by tweaking your diet or adding a short walk to your routine, and gradually build up. Remember, the goal is to support your gut-brain axis for a healthier, happier aging process. It's never too late to start making changes to improve your quality of life as you age.

CASE STUDIES

Let's delve into some transformative gut health stories experienced by older people. Through these, it becomes evident that understanding and nurturing the gut-brain relationship can lead to remarkable improvements in physical and mental well-being.

Take, for instance, the story of Margaret, a 72-year-old retiree who had been battling chronic fatigue, mild cognitive impairment, and a general sense of unhappiness for years. Her journey began with a simple shift in her diet, incorporating more fermented foods and a variety of prebiotic-rich vegetables based on advice from her healthcare provider. Over several months, Margaret noticed a significant uplift in her energy levels, a sharper memory, and an overall improvement in her mood. This change was not just in her head; her family and friends remarked on her renewed zest for life. Margaret's story shows the power of dietary adjustments in reversing the signs of aging through the gut-brain axis.

Then there's James, an 80-year-old who had resigned to the idea that his best years were behind him. Suffering from insomnia and depression, James felt disconnected from the world around him. However, after being introduced to the concept of gut health and its impact on mental well-being, James decided to give probiotics a try, alongside engaging in light, regular exercise through bi-weekly tai chi sessions. To his astonishment, within a few weeks, his sleep patterns began to normalize, and his depressive symptoms started to wane. James's transformation highlights the interconnectedness of physical activity, gut health, and mental well-being, especially as we age.

These stories are powerful reminders of the gut-brain axis's role in our overall health and well-being, particularly as we navigate aging. They illustrate that it's never too late to make changes that can transform our quality of life for the better. By embracing the principles of gut health, individuals of all ages can unlock the door to a healthier, happier, and more vibrant existence.

CHAPTER SUMMARY

- Aging affects gut health and the gut-brain axis, influencing mood and cognitive functions.
- Changes in gut microbiota with age can contribute to cognitive decline, mood disorders, and weakened immune systems.
- The gut microbiome's diversity decreases with age, affecting cognitive health and increasing susceptibility to neurodegenerative diseases.
- Factors like diet, lifestyle, medication, and decreased digestive function impact gut microbiota composition.
- Dietary modifications, physical activity, hydration, and stress management can support a healthy gut-brain axis as we get older.
- Nutritional needs for the golden years of life focus on supporting gut health with fiber, hydration, omega-3s, antioxidants, and probiotics.

- Lifestyle adjustments, including diet, exercise, sleep, stress management, and social connections, are crucial for maintaining a healthy gut-brain axis while navigating the practical aspects of aging.

CHAPTER 10
CHRONIC CONDITIONS AND THE GUT-BRAIN CONNECTION

Diving into the intricate world of our gut, we uncover a universe teeming with microorganisms, each playing a pivotal role in our overall health. This chapter peels back the layers of the microbiome's role in chronic illness, revealing a fascinating interplay between our gut flora and long-term health conditions.

It's becoming increasingly clear that disruptions in the gut microbiome – known as dysbiosis – can contribute to various chronic conditions, from autoimmune diseases like rheumatoid arthritis and multiple sclerosis to metabolic disorders like obesity and type 2 diabetes. Even more compelling is the evidence linking gut health to neurological conditions, including Alzheimer's disease and autism spectrum disorders.

But how does this happen? The answer lies in the gut-brain axis, of course. Through a combination of hormonal, immune, and neural pathways, the state of your gut can send ripples across to your brain. Inflammation is a key player here. When your gut is out of balance, it can trigger an inflammatory response that may contribute to the development or exacerbation of chronic illnesses.

The implications of this suggest that nurturing our gut microbiome might improve our digestive health and offer new ways to manage or even prevent chronic conditions. It's a reminder of the old saying, "You are what you eat," but with a modern twist: your health is as much about the microscopic inhabitants of your gut as it is about the food you feed them.

In essence, the microbiome's role in chronic illness demonstrates the interconnectedness of our body systems. It's a complex puzzle, but as we learn more, the path to better health might just run through our gut.

AUTOIMMUNE DISEASES

The gut-brain connection plays a pivotal role in developing and managing autoimmune conditions. It's an intricate and intimate relationship, with each affecting the other in a continuous communication loop.

Imagine a scenario where the body mistakenly turns against itself, with the immune system targeting its own tissues. This is the harsh reality for those living with autoimmune diseases. The gut, home to trillions of good and bad bacteria, becomes a battleground. The balance of this microbial community can sway the immune response, tipping the scales toward inflammation or balance.

Research suggests a leaky gut may allow harmful substances to enter the bloodstream, triggering an immune response. This response can become overzealous, leading to systemic inflammation and, potentially, the onset of autoimmune diseases. Neurotransmitters and hormones produced in the gut can also influence immune function. This demonstrates the gut's role as a key player in immune regulation.

The gut-brain axis presents a novel pathway for intervention in managing autoimmune diseases. Strategies aimed at restoring gut health, such as the use of probiotics, prebiotics, and dietary modifications, offer hope. These approaches seek to rebalance the microbial community, reduce inflammation, and promote immune tolerance.

Fostering a healthy dialogue between the gut and the brain may help us unlock relief for individuals battling autoimmune conditions. Understanding the gut-brain connection can have immense potential for treating and managing such conditions. It challenges us to think differently about health and disease, pushing the boundaries of traditional medicine. It opens new doors to innovative treatments and a deeper understanding of autoimmune conditions.

GASTROINTESTINAL DISORDERS

When we dive into the world of gastrointestinal disorders, we're not just talking about an upset stomach or the occasional heartburn. We're exploring a complex landscape where the gut and the brain communicate in ways we're only beginning to understand. This intricate connection plays a pivotal role in the development and management of various gastrointestinal conditions.

When the gut-brain connection is disrupted and gastrointestinal disorders develop, it's not just the gut that suffers; our mental health can take a hit, too. Conditions like irritable bowel syndrome, Crohn's disease, ulcerative colitis, and even gastroesophageal reflux disease are not just about physical discomfort. They're deeply intertwined with our mental well-being.

Let's return to the feeling of having butterflies in your stomach before a big presentation. That's the gut-brain connection in action. Now, imagine that feeling amplified and constant, affecting your daily life. That's the reality for many people living with gastrointestinal disorders. The stress and anxiety that come with these conditions can exacerbate symptoms, creating a vicious cycle that's hard to break.

But here's the silver lining: understanding this connection sheds light on new possibilities for treatment. Traditional approaches have primarily focused on the physical symptoms, but we're now seeing the benefits of integrating mental health support. Techniques like cognitive-behavioral therapy, mindfulness, and stress management can offer relief. It's about treating the person as a whole, not just the symptoms.

When managing gastrointestinal disorders, it's crucial to remember that the mind and body are not separate entities. They're deeply connected; nurturing this connection can lead to better health outcomes. Whether through dietary changes, mental health support, or a combination of both, the path to relief is holistic. It's a journey of understanding and respecting the intricate dialogue between our gut and brain and harnessing this knowledge for healing.

HOLISTIC MANAGEMENT APPROACHES

When discussing managing chronic conditions, especially those intertwined with the gut-brain connection, it's easy to get lost in the sea of medical jargon and complex treatment plans. But let's take a step back and consider a more holistic approach. It's not just about what pill to take or what food to eat; it's about looking at the whole picture—your lifestyle, environment, and gut health.

So, how can we leverage our understanding of the gut-brain axis to manage chronic conditions? It's crucial to understand that our gut health significantly impacts our overall well-being and mental health. A holistic management plan incorporates diet, stress management techniques, sleep, physical activity, and support - elements we've covered in various chapters of this book.

Managing chronic conditions through the lens of the gut-brain connection is about more than just addressing symptoms. It's about nurturing your body and mind as a whole, recognizing the intricate ways they interact, and making lifestyle changes that support both. This could be done through diet, exercise, sleep, mindfulness and stress management techniques, and other holistic practices discussed in earlier chapters. It's a journey, no doubt, but one worth embarking on.

CASE STUDIES

The stories of those who navigate chronic conditions are as varied as they are enlightening. Let's delve into a few of these, understanding that behind every case is a person's journey toward better health.

First, meet Karen, a middle-aged woman diagnosed with rheumatoid arthritis, an autoimmune condition. The chronic pain and fatigue were overwhelming. Karen's journey took a turn when her healthcare provider suggested exploring the role of gut health in autoimmune diseases. Karen found a new lease on life by adjusting her diet to eliminate inflammatory foods and introducing gut-healing supplements. The changes didn't cure her condition but significantly reduced her symptoms and improved her quality of life. It is a powerful testament to the connection between her gut and immune system.

Next, consider the story of Bec, who suffered from chronic depression. Despite trying various medications, her battle with depression seemed endless. It was only when her therapist introduced the concept of the gut-brain connection that Bec began to explore this concept. By focusing on gut health through diet and probiotics, Bec experienced a noticeable shift in her mood and energy levels. This approach didn't replace her need for therapy and medication but became a valuable component of her overall treatment plan.

These stories reveal a critical message: the gut-brain connection should be considered when managing chronic conditions. While each person's path is unique, the underlying theme is clear—addressing gut health can improve physical and mental health outcomes. It's a reminder that in the complex web of chronic illness, sometimes the answers lie not just in treating symptoms but in understanding and nurturing the intricate connections within our bodies.

CHAPTER SUMMARY

- The microbiome plays a key role in chronic illnesses, and gut health influences a wide range of conditions, including metabolic and neurological disorders.
- The gut-brain connection plays a crucial role in autoimmune diseases. These diseases involve the immune system attacking the body's tissues, and they are influenced by gut microbial balance.
- Dietary changes and focusing on gut health can potentially alter the course of autoimmune diseases.
- Research indicates that a leaky gut may trigger immune responses, leading to autoimmune diseases, with gut-produced neurotransmitters affecting immune function.

- Gastrointestinal disorders are deeply connected to mental well-being, with stress and diet affecting gut health and vice versa.
- Strategies like probiotics, prebiotics, and dietary modifications that restore gut health offer new avenues for managing chronic conditions.

CHAPTER 11
THE FUTURE OF GUT-BRAIN RESEARCH

As we peer into the future of gut-brain research, it's clear that we're on the cusp of some truly groundbreaking discoveries. The field is buzzing with potential, and several emerging trends promise to shape our understanding of how the gut and brain communicate.

One of the most exciting areas of exploration is the role of the gut microbiome in brain development and function. Scientists are beginning to unravel how these microscopic inhabitants of our gut can influence our mood, behavior, and even cognitive abilities. This research is paving the way for new treatments for a range of conditions, including depression, anxiety, and autism spectrum disorders. Imagine a future where probiotics could play a role in managing mental health alongside or even in place of traditional pharmaceuticals.

Another trend gaining momentum is the use of personalized nutrition to support gut-brain health. As we better understand the unique interplay between diet, the microbiome, and the brain, there's a growing interest in tailoring dietary recommendations to individual needs. This personalized approach could revolutionize the way we think about diet and mental health, moving beyond one-size-fits-all advice to strategies that are finely tuned to each person's biology.

Technological advancements are also set to transform gut-brain research. Wearable devices and smart technology are making it easier than ever to monitor gut health and its impact on the brain in real time. This data could unlock new insights into the complex relationship between our gut and our brain, leading to more effective interventions and therapies.

Finally, there's a growing recognition of the importance of a holistic approach to gut-brain health. Researchers and clinicians are increasingly looking at the big picture, considering factors like stress, sleep, and exercise in their studies. This holistic perspective acknowledges that many factors influence gut-brain health, and addressing it requires a comprehensive, integrated approach.

As we look to the future, it's clear that the journey of understanding the gut-brain connection is far from over. With each new discovery, we're not only unraveling the mysteries of the human body but also opening up new possibilities for health and well-being. The road ahead is filled with promise, and I, for one, can't wait to see where it leads.

INNOVATIVE RESEARCH METHODS

New, innovative research methods promise to deepen our understanding of the gut-brain relationship. The exploration of the gut-brain axis is moving beyond traditional studies, embracing cutting-edge technologies and interdisciplinary approaches that could revolutionize how we think about mental and physical health.

One of the most exciting developments is the use of big data analytics and machine learning. Researchers are now able to sift through vast amounts of data from diverse sources, including genetic information, dietary patterns, and even social media usage, to uncover patterns and correlations that were previously invisible. This holistic approach allows for a more nuanced understanding of how various factors influence the gut-brain connection, potentially leading to personalized treatment plans that are tailored to an individual's unique biological and lifestyle profile.

Another groundbreaking method is the use of organoids, sometimes referred to as "mini-brains" or "mini-guts," grown in the lab from stem cells. These organoids can mimic the structure and function of human organs, providing a powerful tool for studying the gut-brain axis in a controlled environment. By observing how these mini-organs interact, scientists can gain insights into the mechanisms at play in neurodegenerative diseases, psychiatric disorders, and beyond, all without the ethical and practical complications of human or animal testing.

Neuroimaging techniques, too, are becoming more sophisticated, offering unprecedented views of the brain in action. Functional magnetic resonance imaging (fMRI) and positron emission tomography (PET) scans can now show how changes in the gut microbiota affect brain activity in real time. This opens up new pathways for understanding how diet, probiotics, and other interventions can influence mental health and cognitive function.

Moreover, the integration of traditional knowledge and modern science is beginning to take center stage. Researchers are increasingly looking to ancient practices, such as Ayurveda and traditional Chinese medicine, for clues about the gut-brain connection that modern science might have overlooked. This fusion of old and new perspectives not only enriches the research landscape but also paves the way for more holistic and integrative approaches to health and wellness.

As we stand on the brink of these exciting advancements, it's clear that the future of gut-brain research holds limitless potential. The innovative research methods being developed today are not just expanding our knowledge of the gut-brain axis; they are reshaping our very approach to health, promising a future where mental and physical well-being are more closely aligned than ever before. The journey ahead is sure to be filled with discoveries that challenge our assumptions and inspire new ways of thinking about the intricate dance between our guts and our brains.

POTENTIAL BREAKTHROUGHS

The promise of potential breakthroughs in gut-brain research sparks a sense of excitement and curiosity. Imagine a future where understanding the intricate dance between our gut and brain could unlock new doors to treating mental health disorders, enhancing cognitive function, and even preventing diseases before they start. This isn't just wishful thinking; it's a real possibility that researchers around the globe are diligently working towards.

One of the most thrilling prospects lies in the development of personalized medicine. Picture a scenario where, based on the unique composition of your gut microbiota, doctors could tailor treatments and dietary recommendations specifically for you. This approach could revolutionize not only how we treat existing conditions but also how we prevent them. The idea that a simple stool sample could provide insights into your mental health and cognitive abilities is no longer far-fetched.

Another potential breakthrough is the discovery of new probiotic strains with specific health benefits. As we deepen our understanding of how different bacteria influence our brain function, we could see the emergence of targeted probiotic supplements designed to enhance mood, improve memory, or even alleviate symptoms of anxiety and depression. These advancements could offer a natural and side-effect-free alternative to traditional pharmaceuticals.

Exploring the gut-brain axis could also lead to innovative therapies for neurodegenerative diseases. Research is already hinting at connections between gut health and conditions like Alzheimer's and Parkinson's. In the future, we might see treatments that focus on altering the gut microbiome to slow down or even reverse the progression of these diseases.

The potential for breakthroughs extends beyond treatment to the realm of diagnostics. Technological advances could enable the development of non-invasive tests to monitor gut-brain health. Imagine a wearable device that tracks changes in your microbiome and alerts you to potential health issues before they become serious. This could empower individuals to take proactive steps toward maintaining their mental and physical well-being.

As we stand on the cusp of these potential breakthroughs, it's clear that the future of gut-brain research holds immense promise. The journey ahead is filled with challenges, but the rewards could be transformative, reshaping our approach to health and wellness in powerful ways. Exploring the gut-brain connection is more than just a scientific endeavor; it's a journey toward understanding the very essence of what it means to be human.

THE ROLE OF TECHNOLOGY

As we delve into the role of technology in the future of gut-brain research, it's clear that we're standing on the brink of a revolution. Imagine a world where your smartphone could help manage your mental health by monitoring your gut microbiome. It sounds like science fiction, right? Yet, thanks to the rapid advancements in technology, this is where we're headed.

Wearable devices, once used primarily for tracking steps and heart rates, are evolving. Researchers are now developing gadgets capable of analyzing sweat, breath, and even the composition of our gut flora. These devices, equipped with sensors that detect changes in our microbiome, could alert us to potential imbalances that affect our mental well-being.

But it's not just wearables that are transforming the landscape. Artificial intelligence (AI) and machine learning are playing pivotal roles in deciphering the complex interactions between the gut and the brain. By sifting through vast amounts of data, AI can identify patterns and connections that would take humans years to uncover. This could lead to personalized dietary recommendations designed to improve both gut health and mental health.

Virtual reality (VR) is emerging as a powerful tool for stress management and mental health therapy. Imagine donning a VR headset to transport yourself to a tranquil forest or a serene beach, all while your gut health is being optimized through guided meditation and stress-reduction exercises. This combination of technology and therapy could offer new avenues for treating conditions linked to the gut-brain axis.

Telemedicine, too, is making it easier for individuals to access care. With the ability to consult healthcare professionals from the comfort of home, people can receive advice on diet, probiotics, and lifestyle changes that support a healthy gut-brain connection. This is particularly beneficial for those living in remote areas or with mobility issues.

The future of gut-brain research is not just about understanding the connection; it's about harnessing technology to improve it. From wearables and AI to VR and telemedicine, technology is set to play a crucial role in advancing our knowledge and treatment of the gut-brain axis. As we continue to explore this fascinating frontier, one thing is clear: the possibilities are as vast as our imagination.

ETHICAL CONSIDERATIONS

As we venture into the uncharted territories of gut-brain research, the excitement is palpable. The potential to unlock new treatments for mental health, improve our understanding of digestive disorders, and even revolutionize our approach to nutrition is within our grasp. However, with great power comes great responsibility. The ethical considerations of this burgeoning field are as complex as they are critical.

First and foremost, privacy concerns stand at the forefront. The intimate nature of gut microbiome data means that researchers must tread carefully to protect individual privacy. Imagine, for a moment, your entire dietary habits, health status, and even aspects of your mental well-being being deciphered from a simple stool sample. The implications for insurance, employment, and personal privacy are profound. Ensuring that this information is safeguarded is not just a courtesy; it's a necessity.

Then there's the matter of consent. As we delve deeper into the gut-brain connection, the subjects of our studies aren't just numbers on a page; they're people with rights and autonomy. Informed consent becomes a labyrinthine process when dealing with the complexities of gut-brain research. Participants must fully understand what they're consenting to, including how their data will be used, the potential risks involved, and the implications of the research findings on their lives.

The potential for misuse of this research must also be addressed. The idea that dietary interventions or microbiome manipulations could alter behavior or mood opens up a Pandora's box of ethical dilemmas. From the perspective of personal autonomy, the line between treatment and manipulation can become dangerously blurred. It's essential that as we forge ahead, we remain vigilant against the commodification of gut-brain interventions as quick fixes for deeper societal issues.

Accessibility and equity also play pivotal roles in the ethical landscape. The benefits of gut-brain research must be available to all, not just those who can afford cutting-edge treatments. This means advocating for policies that ensure equitable access to any breakthroughs. The goal is to uplift, not to widen, existing health disparities.

In conclusion, the path forward in gut-brain research is fraught with ethical challenges, but it's a path worth taking. By approaching these issues with integrity, transparency, and a commitment to equity, we can navigate the ethical minefield and emerge on the other side with discoveries that have the power to transform lives. The future of gut-brain research is not just about what we can do but what we should do. And that's a journey we must embark on with our eyes wide open.

GLOBAL PERSPECTIVES

As we cast our gaze across the globe, it's clear that the future of gut-brain research is not just a matter of scientific curiosity but a burgeoning field that holds the promise of revolutionizing how we understand and treat a myriad of health conditions. From the bustling research labs of North America to the ancient medicinal practices of Asia, the exploration of the gut-brain connection is a vivid tapestry of global collaboration and innovation.

In Europe, for instance, researchers are delving deep into the genetic markers that might link gut health to mental well-being, offering a glimpse into personalized medicine that could tailor treatments to the individual's unique genetic makeup. Meanwhile, in Asia, the integration of traditional herbal remedies with cutting-edge microbiome research is opening new pathways for holistic approaches to mental health.

Africa, with its rich biodiversity, is a treasure trove of yet-to-be-discovered microbes that could play a pivotal role in gut-brain health. Scientists and traditional healers alike are beginning to collaborate more closely, recognizing that the wisdom of ancient practices and the precision of modern science can complement each other beautifully.

Down under in Australia, researchers are focusing on the environmental impacts on gut health, studying everything from the effects of urban living to the potential benefits of rural microbes. This research is crucial in understanding how our changing world is affecting our health, from our guts to our brains.

Across the Americas, there's a growing emphasis on the societal and economic factors that influence gut health, such as diet, stress, and access to healthcare. This holistic view acknowledges that the gut-brain connection is not just a matter of biology but is deeply influenced by the broader context of our lives.

What's truly exciting is the way technology is knitting these diverse strands of research together. Digital health platforms, artificial intelligence, and big data analytics are enabling researchers to share findings, collaborate on projects, and analyze vast amounts of data like never before. This global network of knowledge is accelerating our understanding of the gut-brain axis at an unprecedented pace.

It's clear that the journey of gut-brain research transcends borders and disciplines. It's a global endeavor that holds the promise of not just better health outcomes but a deeper understanding of the intricate connections that make us human. The path ahead is as vast as it is exciting, and it's a journey we're all on together, each of us playing a part in unraveling the intricacies of the gut-brain connection.

CHAPTER SUMMARY

- The future of gut-brain research is poised for groundbreaking discoveries, particularly in how the gut microbiome influences brain development, mood, and behavior. This could potentially lead to new treatments for mental health conditions.
- Personalized nutrition is emerging as a key trend. Dietary recommendations are being tailored to individual gut-brain health needs, moving beyond generic advice.
- Technological advancements, including wearable devices and artificial intelligence, are transforming research by enabling real-time monitoring of gut health and its impact on the brain.
- Innovative research methods, such as big data analytics, organoids, and neuroimaging, are deepening our understanding of the gut-brain axis and paving the way for personalized medicine.
- Potential breakthroughs include personalized medicine based on gut microbiota, new probiotic strains for mental health, and non-invasive diagnostics for gut-brain health monitoring.
- As the field advances, ethical considerations, including privacy, consent, accessibility, and environmental impact, are critical and should be carefully considered.

THE ROAD AHEAD

It's hard not to feel a sense of awe as we stand at the threshold of what feels like a new era in understanding the intricate relationship between our gut and brain. The journey through the pages of this book has been nothing short of a revelation, peeling back layer after layer of complexity and connection that defines the human experience in ways we're only beginning to understand.

Reflecting on the journey, it's clear that the gut-brain connection is not just a fascinating scientific story; it's a deeply personal one. Each discovery, each piece of evidence, and each story shared in these chapters underscores a truth that feels both ancient and newly discovered: we are holistic beings, and our health cannot be compartmentalized.

The science of the gut-brain connection is about more than just neurotransmitters, hormones, or even the microbiome itself. It's about what we eat, how we move, the quality of our sleep, and the ways we manage stress. All of these factors influence our physical health and mental and emotional well-being.

It's about recognizing that our bodies and minds are not separate entities but are deeply and intricately linked.

Perhaps the most powerful takeaway is the sense of empowerment that comes with this knowledge. Understanding the gut-brain axis gives us a new lens through which to view our health and well-being. It offers us new strategies for nurturing our mental health through gut health, enhancing our physical health by attending to our emotional well-being, and finding balance in our lives through a holistic approach to health.

As we look at the road ahead, it's clear that the journey is far from over. The field of gut-brain research is burgeoning, with discoveries and innovations on the horizon that promise to deepen our understanding even further. But even as we eagerly anticipate these breakthroughs, there's much we can do now to harness the power of the gut-brain connection in our own lives.

The future of gut-brain health is not just in the hands of scientists and researchers; it's in ours, too. It's in the choices we make every day, in our diet and exercise, how we manage stress and the importance we place on our sleep and emotional well-being.

So, let's carry forward the insights and lessons learned. Let's approach our health and well-being with curiosity, compassion, and a renewed connection to the intricate systems that make us who we are. The road ahead is promising, and it's ours to travel with intention, curiosity, and hope.

MONITORING PROGRESS AND LONG-TERM SUSTAINABILITY

As you continue on your journey to discover and explore your gut health, monitoring progress and making adjustments is not just a recommendation but a necessity.

Let's start with the basics: keeping a journal. This might

sound old school, but trust me, it's your compass in this journey. You could do this in a notebook or using an app on your phone. Every day, jot down what you eat, how you feel physically and emotionally, your exercise routine, and the quality of your sleep. Over time, patterns will emerge. You might notice that certain foods trigger bloating or mood swings or that physical activity enhances your digestion and mental clarity. This journal becomes your map, guiding your next steps.

Now, onto the adjustments. They're not just about cutting out the bad stuff; it's also about introducing and experimenting with the good. Found that dairy doesn't agree with you? Explore the world of plant-based alternatives. Have you realized that a brisk walk in the morning boosts your mood for the day? Make it a non-negotiable part of your routine. The key here is gradual, sustainable change. Rome wasn't built in a day, and neither is a healthy gut.

Remember that this journey is uniquely yours. What works for someone else might not work for you, and that's okay. The goal is to find your equilibrium, where your gut health supports your overall well-being, allowing you to live your life to the fullest. So, keep monitoring, adjusting, and moving forward. The journey to better health is a marathon, not a sprint, and every step forward is a victory.

Embracing a gut-healthy lifestyle is akin to planting a garden. Initially, it demands effort, patience, and trial and error. But with time, as you nurture it, it blossoms, rewarding you with vibrant health and a deeper connection between your gut and brain. The key to this flourishing relationship lies in long-term sustainability. It's about making choices you can stick with over the years, not just for a few weeks or months.

Long-term sustainability in nurturing the gut-brain connection is about integrating these changes into your life in a manageable and enjoyable way. It's a journey of discovery, learning what works best for you, and adapting as your needs and circumstances change. The goal is not just to live longer but to live better with a healthy gut and sharp mind. So, take it one step at a time, be kind to yourself. Your gut and brain will thank you for it.

SEEKING SUPPORT

Support comes in many forms. It could be a family member who decides to embark on this lifestyle change with you, making it easier to plan meals and activities that benefit your gut health. It could be a healthcare professional, like a nutritionist or a therapist, who provides guidance tailored to your needs. Or it could be the stories of others who have seen remarkable changes in their health, inspiring you to stick with your new habits even when it gets tough.

One of the most beautiful aspects of seeking out community and support is the ripple effect it creates. As you learn and grow, you become a beacon of knowledge and encouragement for others. Your successes and challenges become lessons for your community, and together, you build a wealth of collective wisdom that can guide newcomers.

Changing long-standing habits can be challenging. There will be days when your motivation wanes. Having a support system provides a safety net for those moments, offering encouragement and reminding you of why you started this journey in the first place.

While the journey to better gut health starts with individual choices, it flourishes with the support of a community. Whether sharing a success story, a setback, or a new discovery, every interaction enriches your journey. So, as you embark on this path, remember to reach out, connect, and build your support network. After all, the journey is not just about reaching the destination but about the camaraderie and insights gained along the way.

STAYING INFORMED AND ENGAGED

The landscape of gut-brain research is evolving rapidly, with discoveries and insights emerging at a pace that can sometimes feel overwhelming. Yet, staying informed and engaged with these advancements is not just beneficial—it's essential for anyone looking to harness the power of their gut to improve mental and physical health.

The question then becomes: How do we stay abreast of the latest findings without getting lost in the sea of information? First and foremost, it's about finding reliable sources. Scientific journals, reputable health websites, and gut health and neuroscience conferences are gold mines of information. Subscribing to newsletters from leading research institutions can also give you a summary of the latest developments.

But it's not just about passive information consumption. Engaging with online and offline communities that share your interest in the gut-brain connection can enrich your understanding and provide support as you apply new knowledge to your life. Forums, social media groups, and local meetups can be invaluable resources for exchanging tips, sharing experiences, and discussing the latest research with like-minded individuals.

Remember, the journey to understanding and optimizing our gut-brain connection is ongoing. As we've explored throughout this book, there's always more to learn. The field is dynamic, and what we understand today may evolve tomorrow. That's why staying curious, open-minded, and proactive about learning is crucial.

Ultimately, the most powerful tool at our disposal is our

body and mind. Listening to our gut, quite literally, can provide us with insights into our health and well-being. As we move forward, let's commit to staying informed, engaged, and connected—not just with the global community of researchers and enthusiasts but with our inner ecosystem. The road ahead is promising; together, we can navigate it with knowledge, understanding, and a sense of shared discovery.

THE CONTINUING EVOLUTION OF GUT-BRAIN RESEARCH

As we stand on the precipice of the future, gazing into the vast expanse of possibilities, the journey of understanding the gut-brain connection is far from over. It's evolving at an unprecedented pace, promising to unravel mysteries that have perplexed humanity for ages. The road ahead is not just an extension of our path; it's an invitation to explore new horizons, challenge the boundaries of our knowledge, and embrace the unknown with open arms.

The continuing evolution of gut-brain research is a testament to human curiosity and resilience. It's a field that refuses to stay static, driven by an insatiable quest for knowledge. Every discovery opens the door to many questions, each more intriguing than the last. What we know today is just a drop in the ocean of what remains to be discovered. The complexity of the gut-brain axis, with its intricate web of neurotransmitters, hormones, and microbes, is a puzzle that we've only just begun to piece together.

In the years to come, we can expect to see groundbreaking research that pushes the boundaries of what we thought was possible. Imagine a world where mental health is managed not only through traditional means but is also influenced by our understanding of the gut-brain axis, where dietary interventions and gut microbiome modulation become standard practice in preventing and treating neurological disorders. This is not just a hopeful vision of the future. It's a genuine possibility based on the trajectory of current research.

Technological advancements will play a pivotal role in this journey. Cutting-edge tools and techniques, some of which are in their infancy today, will enable researchers to explore the gut-brain axis with greater precision and depth. From sophisticated imaging technologies to advanced genetic sequencing, the arsenal of tools at our disposal is expanding, bringing us closer to unlocking the secrets of the gut-brain connection.

However, the road ahead is not without its challenges. The complexity of the gut-brain axis means that research in this field is like navigating a labyrinth, where each turn can lead to unexpected discoveries or dead ends. Collaboration across disciplines will be crucial. Neuroscientists, microbiologists, nutritionists, and psychologists, among others, must join forces, sharing insights and perspectives to build a holistic understanding of the gut-brain connection.

As we embark on this exciting journey into the future, one thing is clear: the potential for improving human health and well-being is immense. The gut-brain connection is a powerful reminder of the interconnectedness of our bodies and minds. The research in this field has the potential to revolutionize the way we think about health, disease, and treatment.

The road ahead is rich with possibility, and the continuing evolution of gut-brain research is a journey that promises to be as fascinating as it is transformative. The future is bright, and it's ours to explore.

THE FUTURE OF HEALTH AND WELLNESS

The intricate dialogue between our digestive system and brain has unveiled a new paradigm in approaching health, emphasizing the importance of a holistic view. As we envision it, the future is not just about treating symptoms but nurturing a harmonious relationship between all aspects of our being.

Imagine a world where personalized nutrition plans based on gut microbiome analysis become the norm, not the exception. In this future, food is not just fuel but medicine, tailored to the unique needs of each individual, preventing diseases before they even take root. The role of probiotics and prebiotics will evolve beyond supplements, becoming integral components of our daily diet, designed to support a diverse and resilient microbiome.

The mental health landscape is poised for a revolution, too. As we unravel the complex interactions between gut health and mental well-being, new treatments for conditions like depression and anxiety will emerge, treatments that target the gut to heal the mind. This could redefine our approach to mental health, moving from a solely pharmaceutical model to one that incorporates dietary changes, stress management techniques, and perhaps even targeted microbiome therapies.

In the realm of research, the future holds the promise of even more sophisticated tools and technologies. Imagine AI-driven platforms that can analyze vast amounts of data to uncover previously hidden connections between diet, microbiome composition, and health outcomes. These insights could lead to breakthroughs in preventing and treating not just gastrointestinal diseases but a wide range of conditions, from autoimmune disorders to neurodegenerative diseases.

Education will also play a pivotal role in this future. As knowledge about the gut-brain connection continues to grow, so will the need to disseminate this information widely. Schools, workplaces, and communities will become hubs of learning, where practical advice on nurturing gut health will be as commonplace as tips on maintaining good hygiene.

Yet, for all the optimism, challenges remain. The complexity of the gut-brain axis means that there are no one-size-fits-all solutions. Navigating the vast sea of information, some of it contradictory, can be daunting for many. Access to the benefits of this knowledge must be equitable, ensuring that advancements in gut-brain health are available to all, not just a privileged few.

As we look to the future, understanding and leveraging the gut-brain connection promises to transform our approach to health and wellness and redefine our very notions of what it means to live a healthy life. Together, step by step, we can move towards a future where the harmony between our gut and our brain paves the way for unparalleled well-being.

FINAL THOUGHTS

As we draw the curtains on this exploration of the gut-brain connection, take a moment to pause and reflect on the journey we've embarked upon together. It has been nothing short of revelatory.

In a world where the pace of scientific discovery accelerates by the day, it's crucial to stay curious and open-minded. The gut-brain axis, a once-obscure area of study, now stands at the forefront of a health revolution, promising insights that could transform our approach to mental and physical well-being.

I remember the first time I stumbled upon the concept of the gut-brain connection. It was during a casual dinner conversation with a friend who, at the time, was navigating the challenges of managing her anxiety. She mentioned how altering her diet and focusing on gut health had led to noticeable improvements in her mental state. This anecdote, simple as it may seem, sparked a curiosity in me that eventually led to the writing of this book. It's a testament to the power of personal stories in driving scientific curiosity and discovery.

As we look to the future, it's clear that the exploration of the gut-brain connection is far from over. With each study, we peel back another layer, revealing more about this complex interplay and its potential to influence everything from our mood to our susceptibility to various diseases. The road ahead is paved with questions yet to be answered, therapies yet to be discovered, and stories yet to be told.

But the journey doesn't end with the closing of this book. It continues in the choices we make every day, from the foods we eat to the way we manage stress and prioritize our mental health. By embracing a holistic view of health that acknowledges the gut-brain connection, we step into a future where well-being is not just about the absence of disease but about the presence of vitality and joy.

I encourage you to keep exploring, questioning, and connecting the dots in your health journey as we part ways. The relationship between our gut and brain is a beautiful reminder of the body's complexity and interconnectedness. It's a reminder that, in the pursuit of health, every piece matters, and every step counts.

YOUR FEEDBACK MATTERS

As we reach the end of this book, I extend my heartfelt gratitude for your time and engagement. It's been an honor to share this journey with you, and I hope it has been as enriching for you as it has been for me.

Your feedback helps me as an independent author and guides fellow readers searching for their next meaningful read. Your insights and reflections are invaluable to me. By sharing them, you contribute to a larger conversation that extends far beyond the pages of this book.

If the ideas we've explored have sparked new thoughts, inspired change, or provided comfort, I'd really appreciate it if you could share your experience with others by leaving a review on the platform on which you purchased this book. Alternatively, you can follow the QR code below.

Thank you once again for your company on this literary adventure. May the insights you've gained stay with you, and may your quest for knowledge be ever-fulfilling.

ABOUT THE AUTHOR

Natasha Harlow is an author and passionate advocate in the field of gut health. She has an academic background in nutritional science and years of research in gut microbiology. Natasha's work is driven by a deep-seated belief in the power of holistic health approaches, and she has dedicated her career to exploring the complex interplay between what we eat and how we feel, think, and behave.

Through her books, Natasha aims to bridge the gap between scientific research and everyday wellness practices, making the intricate details of gut health accessible and actionable for everyone. Her writing not only sheds light on the latest findings in the field but also offers practical advice for nurturing a healthy gut. She inspires readers to take control of their wellbeing by understanding the foundational role of gut health in overall vitality.

Printed in Dunstable, United Kingdom